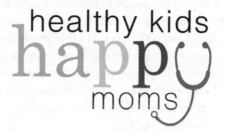

"I know Dr. Kilbane well. She possesses a unique blend of smarts, heart, and passion that together give substance to her life's work: improving the lives of children and their families, with a laser focus on nutrition. Readers of *Healthy Kids, Happy Moms* will access a clear guide for raising healthy children, one supported by research and experience, providing important information only rarely touched upon during a traditional time-constrained doctor's visit. Dr. Kilbane's program is credible and actionable and can help set the stage for children to become optimally well. That makes for a happy kid as well as a happy mom (and dad)."

—RUSSELL H. GREENFIELD, MD
Graduate of the first class at the Andrew Weil Center for
Integrative Medicine, University of Arizona College of
Medicine; Clinician and Consultant attending to individual,
community, and employee health and healing

"When I met Dr. Kilbane and learned about her work, the first words out of my mouth were: 'Where were you when my boys were young?' They struggled with many of the issues this book helps improve or, in some cases, resolve altogether. She has become a leader in the field of pediatric health and nutrition. Her program is proactive toward your child's health. She doesn't take the all-too-common 'wait and see' approach that I grew so frustrated with when my boys were little. If you're ready to stop the cycle of recurrent illnesses or get on track to a healthier diet and lifestyle with your child and family, this book is for you!"

—JJ VIRGIN
Four-time *New York Times* Bestselling Author, Celebrity
Nutritionist, and Fitness Expert

"I have known Dr. Kilbane for years. We both completed our integrative medical training with Andrew Weil, MD. On behalf of children, she has forged a new path in the field of integrative pediatric health. I have relied on her expertise and care for my own child, with outstanding results. There is usually not one 'magic bullet' to heal a child. That's why Dr. Kilbane's comprehensive program is so powerful. It offers the step-by-step approach she uses in her clinic. To have this information at your fingertips could be a game-changer for your child and family, if you're willing to take the time and make some not always easy—but very doable—changes. I highly recommend this book, both personally and professionally, for all parents and pediatric healthcare practitioners seeking to understand how to stop the cycle of recurrent illnesses in children."

—JEFF GLADD, MD
National Speaker and Leader on patient empowerment,
lifestyle-based healthcare, and technology integration into
private practice; Medical Director, GladdMD; Chief Medical
Officer, Fullscript

•

"I'm so grateful for Dr. Kilbane and her work to restore the health of our children! I am one of the fortunate parents who has been able to have Dr. Kilbane as an advisor to support my son, and she offers one-of-a-kind solutions that really work! No more trying things that only waste your time and money, and leave your poor baby still sick. I am super excited that these same solutions are now available to parents all over the world. This book is practical, is research-based, and provides a clear strategy to resolve common childhood ailments and to help children thrive the way they are meant to. She has taken into account the physiology and biochemistry of a child's system and, with her years of clinical experience, has created a new paradigm for children's healthcare. This book can help you gain peace of mind about your child's health and allow you to take a break from being Dr. Mom and spending many late nights on Dr. Google, so you can enjoy the precious time you have together."

—IZABELLA WENTZ, PHARMD
Mama, Pharmacist, and *New York Times*
Bestselling Author of *Hashimoto's Protocol*

•

"Dr. Sheila's approach to nutrition for our children is refreshing and doable, but most importantly it's healing and wholesome."

—JEN HANSARD
Bestselling Author of *Simple Green
Smoothies & Simple Green Meals*

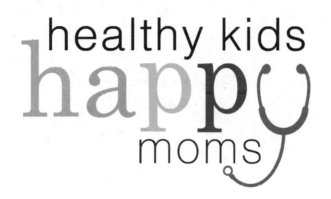

healthy kids
happy
moms

healthy kids
happy
moms

**7 Steps to Heal and Prevent
Common Childhood Illnesses**

SHEILA KILBANE, MD

with Tamela Rich

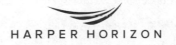

HARPER HORIZON

ISBN 978-0-7852-4107-2 (eBook)

ISBN 978-0-7852-4106-5 (HC)

Library of Congress Control Number: 2021936762

Printed in Canada

21 22 23 24 25   TC   10 9 8 7 6 5 4 3 2 1

To Susan and Kit

I miss you both every day.

My two dear friends here in Charlotte passed away
during the writing of this book.

My hope for the words on these pages is that they allow you,
the reader, to feel seen, heard, and understood—
the way Susan and Kit made me feel.

Feeling heard is where true healing begins.

contents

foreword

HEALTHY KIDS, HAPPY MOMS promises to help millions of children in need. Written by a board-certified pediatrician who is also trained in nutrition and integrative medicine, Dr. Kilbane's accurate nutrition information, along with clear, step-by-step guidance, makes this book an important asset for parents and healthcare practitioners.

Diet of poor quality is the single leading cause of chronic disease and premature death in the modern world. That harm begins early in life, and early in life is the best time to turn things around. Dr. Kilbane is right to focus on "fixing" broken diets in childhood and at the level of family.

Getting diet right is not about satisfying someone else's standard or ticking off a box. Food plays a significant role in our inflammatory responses. Excess, chronic inflammation doesn't allow the immune system or, for that matter, any organ-system of the body, to work optimally. The most vulnerable among us suffer the gravest consequences from poor food quality. High levels of added sugar, refined carbohydrates, and ultraprocessed foods are the least expensive and most readily available to our children. These foods are aggressively marketed as well, essentially propagating profit at the expense of our children's health. Dr. Kilbane and I agree emphatically: This has to stop!

Empowered with the information here, you can be part of that overdue remedy. *Healthy Kids, Happy Moms* is practical, actionable, and easy to understand. Dr. Kilbane blends the science of food and physiology with simple explanations and clarifying graphics. Clear, expert guidance here can help drown out the distracting din of marketing messages that sell our children and families the synthetic food that makes so many of us sick.

Diet and exercise habits learned while young will stick throughout life, and vitality is among the greatest of gifts we parents can bestow—a gift that keeps on giving.

Dr. Kilbane's book offers every reader the opportunity to work with a compassionate, integrative pediatrician, right in your own home. This book details the recipe for moving your child from a place of recurrent illness and excess inflammation to one of health. With that health comes joy because, in general, healthy, vital people—kids and adults alike—feel better and have more fun.

At times, we can forget that health isn't the ultimate prize. Health makes living the way we want to live more possible—and that, of course, is the prize.

We cannot control everything our children are exposed to, but we can feed and nurture them in ways that promote health instead of illness and enthusiasm rather than resistance. All children deserve the opportunity to eat healthy, clean, real food. With this book in all the right hands, many more will have it!

—DAVID L. KATZ, MD, MPH

Past President, American College of Lifestyle Medicine
Founding Director, Prevention Research Center, Yale University
President, True Health Initiative

how i stumbled upon the power of nutrition

N 2006, WHEN I was about a year out of residency, I prided myself on the fact that I could manage my pediatric patients' symptoms, whatever they were, with drugs. Laxatives, antihistamines, antacids, steroids (topical, inhaled, oral, or even sprayed into the nose), and antibiotics . . . two, three, and yes, sometimes even four medications. All the while I convinced the parents (and myself) that this was perfectly safe. I prescribed laxatives for years on end and wrote antacid prescriptions for three-month-old babies.

However, when I began medical school, I never imagined my day-to-day life would entail running from room to room, stressed and anxious. I even found myself getting defensive toward parents who continued to ask questions.

The bubble inside my head said, "By the way, this visit is scheduled in a ten-minute slot, and I have been in here for twenty-five minutes, so please—no more questions that I don't have answers for!"

I can't believe I'm admitting this, as those were not some of my finer moments as a pediatrician, whose purpose is to help children. But these challenges catalyzed my desire to seek better ways to help my patients. Either that, or I would have to find a new profession.

The question that came over and over from these moms was, "Isn't there another way?"

I had no idea at that time that nutrition played such a significant role in chronic and recurrent childhood illnesses. I also had no idea that the medications I was prescribing, along with the inflammatory foods the kids were eating, were holding my patients in a *sick cycle*. The antibiotics, in addition to killing the harmful bacteria in the ears, lungs, or sinus cavities, were also killing the healthy bacteria in their guts. The antacids were preventing them from properly absorbing proteins and other nutrients such as vitamin B_{12}, and the laxatives were a Band-Aid for their constipation. Kids don't have laxative deficiencies, so why do so many kids need to take a daily laxative to have a bowel movement? All of these medications treated the symptoms (and are absolutely needed at times), but this way of practicing didn't force me to dig deeper and understand what was driving these illnesses.

The kids I saw repeatedly were the ones who were struggling with one or more of the many common childhood illnesses. I got to know these families well because they were in the office almost once a month. These conditions tend to flare up regularly, and unless we identify and treat the underlying triggers, they continue to recur:

- Colic
- Reflux
- Eczema
- Keratosis pilaris (bumps on the back of the arms, cheeks, or thighs)
- Recurrent ear and sinus infections
- Chronic runny nose
- Allergies
- Asthma
- Stomach aches
- Constipation or loose stools

I remember my *aha* moment about food and children's health like it was yesterday . . .

CASE STUDY

JOHNNY

SYMPTOMS: ECZEMA AND RECURRENT EAR INFECTIONS

Johnny was a sweet baby boy I'd been seeing since he was born. He was a precious child with blue eyes, short brown hair, and pink cheeks that were more itchy than rosy. Eczema, which had started shortly after birth, covered his body. Recurrent ear infections, which started around five months of age, caused fussiness. He'd already required several rounds of antibiotics for ear infections, as well as steroid cream to control the eczema. His mother was always wondering if we could be doing something else to help him.

At his nine-month wellness visit, Johnny's mother told me, "I took dairy out of Johnny's diet since our last visit, and his eczema is almost completely gone." Since mom was breastfeeding, she also removed dairy from her diet, so her breast milk wouldn't expose him to the cow milk protein casein.

"I don't know if it has anything to do with you both being off dairy, but go ahead and stay off it, and I'll figure out how we're going to get calcium, fat, and vitamin D into both of you," I said.

Though the eczema was much improved, it hadn't fully resolved. Furthermore, at Johnny's ten- and eleven-month visits, he still had fluid behind both of his eardrums. Persistent residual fluid is a well-known complication of ear infections and, if left untreated, can lead to hearing impairment. I referred Johnny to an ear, nose, and throat doctor to be evaluated for ear tubes, and his surgery was scheduled.

His one-year well visit was on a Monday. The Sunday prior to this visit, Johnny's mother ate a big omelet, and he had a huge flare-up of his eczema. We decided to ditch eggs *and* dairy from Johnny's diet and mom's diet, but we still planned on the ear tube surgery to protect his hearing.

Then, due to an insurance glitch, Mom postponed the surgery.

A month after that one-year well visit, the surgery hadn't been rescheduled, and they came to have his ears rechecked.

I expected the usual: little Johnny with a few remnant dry, itchy eczema patches on his elbows, knees, and trunk and fluid in his ears.

But the usual isn't what I found that day.

The eczema had *completely* cleared up. And the fluid behind his eardrums? *Nowhere to be found.*

A disco ball dropped down from the clinic ceiling, and Johnny's mother and I did a happy dance. We could skip the stress, expense, and nerve-wracking experience of watching a baby get wheeled into surgery. He also wouldn't have general anesthesia, which, while safe, always carries some risk.

I couldn't deny what I was seeing, but I couldn't explain it either. Was food playing a role? As he'd gotten older, had time resolved his eczema and ear infections? Was it all coincidence?

Over the next seven months, I observed Johnny's ears and skin. As long as mom kept eggs and dairy out of his diet, his skin and ear issues didn't return. By listening to Johnny's mother and putting these pieces together, we prevented further rounds of antibiotics and topical steroids.

When I saw this same scenario play out with hundreds of other patients, I realized it was more than coincidence. The connection among nutrition, health, and inflammation (which I explain in this book) isn't something I learned in medical school or pediatric training (circa 2000), nor did many other doctors. Medical schools don't teach students how to follow the threads of common childhood illnesses to their root cause. Rather, they teach doctors to use medications to treat each illness, how to prescribe these medications, and how to assess their effectiveness.

And where has this approach gotten us? Fifty percent of American children suffer from chronic illnesses—more than at any other time in our history. Chronic childhood illnesses have gone from being a rarity to being the norm.

AMERICAN MEDICINE HAS A LOT TO LEARN

The United States has some of the best-trained doctors and the most sophisticated medical technology on the planet. Yet we're nowhere near the healthiest country. According to a 2014 Commonwealth Fund report, the US ranked last among eleven industrialized countries on measures of health system quality, efficiency, access to care, and equity.[1]

Additionally, in 2011, the US spent the highest amount of money per patient, at $8,508 annually, yet we had the lowest overall outcomes.[2] This is compared to the United Kingdom, which ranked first overall and spent less than half of what the US did per patient, at $3,406 annually.[3]

In another survey of health measurements, by the Organization for Economic Cooperation and Development (OECD), the US ranked twenty-sixth out of thirty-four comparable countries. The OECD report stated:

> The US spends far more than any other comparable country, yet we get far less for our money. Americans are fatter, die younger, and don't get particularly good treatment for many diseases, with the exception of strokes and cancer. We spend 17 percent of our gross domestic product on health care compared to the average of 9.3 for the other countries. We also spend more than the average out-of-pocket for health care. This is just under 3 percent of total household budget, compared to 1.5 percent in Britain, France, and the Netherlands.[4]

I'd love for the healthcare reform discussion to include the food industry, the availability of healthy food to people of all economic levels, and more comprehensive nutrition training in medical schools. These topics also need to be tackled on a policy level. Imagine if growing organic fruits and vegetables became a priority for our government. Imagine if schools were supported to feed our children fresh, healthy food, instead of inflammatory processed foods and sugary drinks. We might not remain the country that spends more on healthcare than any other country in the world, while remaining thirty-seventh in health outcomes. Let's invest more time, money, and effort on the front end of our health on food, nutrition education, and physical activity and less on the back end in medical costs.

LEARNING TO LISTEN

After Johnny's turnaround, I continued to listen to parents when they told me about improvement in their child's illness after a nutrition change, seriously considering the parents' intuition. Then I'd research and investigate reputable studies to determine if any science supported the parents' hypothesis. As I did, the link between food and illness became more and more clear, but it took years for me to wrap my head around how profound this link is. Each time I learned something new I had to figure out how to counsel parents and implement these nutrition changes in a busy pediatric practice. It wasn't enough to tell them what the child should not eat—they also needed to know what the child *should* eat.

In spite of my discoveries, the significant skepticism among medical doctors about nutrition made me keep my findings to myself and my families. One day, a fellow pediatrician said to me, "Sheila, what is that voodoo medicine you're practicing?" I just laughed. But within a year, thanks to rapidly growing research, that same doctor asked me how to dose probiotics for one of his patients.

A SECOND DISCO BALL DROP

I had been utilizing nutrition in my pediatric practice for years before I decided to do a fellowship at the Andrew Weil Center for Integrative Medicine. That's where I, along with sixty-five other healthcare practitioners, learned how every aspect of our environment impacts our health, from what we eat, to how we live, and even what we believe. We commiserated about the difficulty of incorporating the kind of counseling that we needed to do with our patients into the strictures of traditional practices that expected us to minimize time spent on each visit.

Shortly after I began that program in 2010, the seasonal flu was rampant in Charlotte and across much of the globe. Into my office walked Sandra and her daughter Julie. Julie tested positive for the flu. Sandra's son Hasan, a darling boy of eight who is on the autism spectrum was also my patient. After taking care of Julie, I asked Sandra how Hasan was doing. She said he was the only one in the household who wasn't sick. Sandra, her husband, and their other two children all had the flu.

One year prior, Sandra and I worked together to eliminate gluten and dairy from Hasan's diet. She'd also incorporated other anti-inflammatory dietary changes and some high-quality, supportive supplements—a probiotic, a whole food supplement, omega 3 fats in the form of fish oil, and vitamin D in the winter.

"Really. Isn't that amazing?" I said. Then I thought, *Why am I not encouraging this effective anti-inflammatory diet and those same foundational supplements for all of my patients?*

In that moment, the disco ball again dropped down from the clinic ceiling, and the idea for this book was born. My epiphany was that I should be talking to all parents about nutrition for the children I was seeing, not just those who were sick and struggling. The profound impact I could have on the health of many children, simply by educating parents and other healthcare practitioners on how to optimize a child's nutrition and strategically add some key supplements, both boggled my mind and filled me with hope.

I had been recommending a variation of Hasan's regimen with other patients, just not to the same extent. At that time, I didn't have the extensive research knowledge, clinical experience, and practical understanding of the role food played in inflammation—and, in turn, how inflammation prevented the immune system from functioning properly. I also didn't have the time to educate families about food. I knew what the kids shouldn't eat, but figuring out what they *should* eat, and how to counsel families on this, remained a work in progress.

Over the years, hundreds of families have come to me after having spent thousands of dollars on testing, x-rays, procedures, specialist visits, medications, and even surgeries, to no avail. After going through my program, they experience significant improvements— sometimes within a week, sometimes a month, and at other times over six months. After spending years studying and practicing integrative pediatrics, I can finally look parents in the eye, with confidence in my ability to offer a more holistic solution, and say, "*Yes*—there is another way!"

A STEP-BY-STEP GUIDE FOR THE WHOLE FAMILY'S HEALTH

After that insightful day with Hasan's mother and sister, I began to talk to all families about nutrition. One of my goals is to help parents understand that our bodies are ecosystems of cells, tissues, organs, and even microorganisms, working seamlessly to keep the whole body-mind-spirit healthy.

I also recognized the need to create a step-by-step guide for parents to follow because few families have access to an integrative pediatrician. That's why I wrote this book and created an online program called *7 Steps to Healthy Kids, Happy Moms*. The book and online program are educational tools, not replacements for good, old-fashioned, face-to-face pediatric care.

I've helped hundreds of children and families break the cycle of recurrent antibiotic use, missed school days, sleepless nights, emergency room visits, and all the accompanying stress that comes along with having a sick child.

If your child suffers from one of the following illnesses—colic, reflux, recurrent ear and/or sinus infections, eczema, keratosis pilaris (bumps on the back of the arms, cheeks, or thighs), stomachaches, constipation or diarrhea, bloating, extreme gas, abdominal pain, chronic runny nose, mouth breathing, snoring, allergies, or asthma—this book offers the possibility of changing your child's health and quality of life forever.

Other issues that often improve through the HKHM program include poor sleep, mood swings, irritability, anxiety, behavior challenges, meltdowns, focus, and attention. And since I recommend the entire family do the program *together*, you'll experience improved health as well. Parents come back two months after changing their family's diet: their skin is clear, they're jogging again, they've dropped several pounds, and they have an all-around better outlook on life.

This book has been written with great care over several years. I love being able to help parents cease the late-night Dr. Google searches, so you can sleep more soundly. This peace of mind allows room for you to feel joy with your child and family again. How much better is it to be laughing over ridiculous idiosyncrasies and goofy jokes, since you're no longer worried about your child's health?!

Most of all, I want to help your child get back into balance and grow into a healthy adult.

healthy cell,

healthy gut,

healthy child

CHAPTER 1

an integrative approach to pediatric medicine

A S A YOUNG CHILD, I would get really sick two or three times a year. I'd lie on the couch in the family room, with a towel and a bucket, barely able to move. The fevers were so high I couldn't even watch TV. I'd get weak enough that my mother would have to carry me to the bathroom. She and I can't remember exactly what age I was when these fevers started, but we think it was first grade (so I would have been seven years old) and that it happened about four or five times over a two-year period.

I realize in this modern era of medicine at our fingertips, it may sound like my mother was waiting a long time to take me in to be checked. I am the youngest of five, and by the time I came along my mother knew that a viral infection did not need an antibiotic and that, more often than not, our bodies are strong and designed to fight most run-of-the-mill childhood illnesses. She was actually quite diligent with my illness, as you will see.

When this first started happening, day four or five of my fever would inevitably result in a trip to Dr. Nowak's office, which I grew to dread. Dr. Nowak would listen to my heart and lungs and feel the glands in my neck. Then I would get an extremely painful shot of penicillin in my rumpus that felt like he was throwing a dart at a bullseye. He didn't do any testing, just gave me a shot. If you've ever had a shot of penicillin, it feels like cement being injected into your backside. I was scared to death of him, and it didn't help that he never spoke to me directly. However, I always got better within two or three days . . . the beauty of antibiotics.

Dr. Nowak told my mother he didn't think I needed any further testing to figure out what was driving the fevers. But once the recurrent pattern of fevers began to emerge, my mother's gut told her something was triggering them, and we needed to get to the root of the issue. As I was writing the chapter, I called Mar (the name we affectionately call my mother) to talk about this pattern. She said it always happened around the time of an event in our family, like a party for a graduation or something. With five kids, some milestone was always on the horizon. Our house would have been buzzing with friends and relatives getting the house ready and food prepared (not that I was likely doing any of that, but I am sure I was running around with all the melee).

Mar noticed that the fevers seemed to be triggered when my system was run down and taxed (stressed) by external factors. (I am having a chuckle as I write this because the same thing happened to me in high school after my brother and I threw a raging party when my parents were out of town. I stayed up all night cleaning the house and two days later, I had an attack of appendicitis and had to have my appendix removed.) Was it coincidence or cause and effect? Of course I will never know, but I don't think it was solely coincidence.

Back to my fevers and my mother's sleuthing. After about the third episode, Mar started to realize that when these fevers happened, nobody else at home was sick. This became her clue that it wasn't likely a virus. However, Dr. Nowak seemed content to continue giving me injections of penicillin. He never attempted to find the underlying cause and rebuked my mother's attempts to do so.

After about the fourth or fifth episode, she took me to the Cleveland Clinic for further testing—back then they didn't require referrals. As Mar and I talked about this in 2020, we marveled at how she figured it all out. She reminds me a great deal of the incredibly bright and tenacious mothers I see in my practice. How did she even know what type of specialist to take me to or which hospital? As Deb Allen, the amazing pharmacist who works with me—and the mother of teenage triplets—always says in our office, "The mother of a sick child is better than an FBI agent any day of the week at finding answers."

I ended up getting a kidney ultrasound and a VCUG (voiding cysto-urethrogram). My kidney function was fine, but they discovered I had a small area on one kidney with an abnormal appearance. (They also found incidentally that I have four kidneys and four ureters . . . if you ever need a kidney, you know where to come.) My young ears remember it being explained that this area had carried a low-level infection for much of my childhood. When my immune system was run down, I'd get a kidney infection. So, the high fevers were recurrent kidney infections, which can easily end up in sepsis (an overwhelming full-body infection where the organs begin to shut down).

The doctors at the Cleveland Clinic prescribed a six-month course of a low-dose antibiotic, and I've never had a problem since. This is the beauty of conventional medicine and of a mother trusting her instinct. Watching my own parents trust their guts when it came to raising us, I have always trusted the mothers in my practice when they tell me they think there is something else going on with their child that we have not figured out yet. This book is for you mothers who know there may be something else to your child's illness than what seems to meet the eye.

I share my kidney infection story with you for two reasons, one professional and the other personal. First, I am quite certain these experiences with Dr. Nowak are the reason I became a pediatrician. I had no voice in his office and I remember vowing then and there that I would become a doctor and that I would speak directly to the children who came to see me. Today, I include the children in my discussion with their parents and give them a say in the plan if at all possible. Second, personally, my experience with Dr. Nowak taught me never to underestimate the mind of a child and their ability to understand and interpret what is happening around them.

As you'll see in this book, food will certainly help many inflammatory issues and it also helps the immune system to work optimally, but we always have to keep the big picture in mind. From my many years of practicing medicine, I can also guarantee that all the right foods and supplements on the planet would not have healed my recurring kidney infections. I needed a course of antibiotics to resolve each kidney infection I had. And then I needed a less potent antibiotic over that long duration to fully clear the issue.

THE INCREASING PREVALENCE OF CHILDHOOD ILLNESSES

My childhood was spent in a suburb of Cleveland. All the Kilbane kids walked to the public elementary school at the end of our street. All five of us cycled through the same amazing teachers at Erieview Elementary School and my memories there are some of my fondest. Fifth grade was the first time I ever remember noticing any type of illness at school, when my friend Lisa was diagnosed with type 1 diabetes. Lisa had to prick her finger at lunch and carry a snack with her at all times.

Think about that: One kid in a school of three hundred had a chronic illness (at least as far as I knew). We didn't have kids using albuterol inhalers or storing EpiPens in the nurse's office in case they got an accidental food exposure. We didn't have peanut-free classrooms or restrictions on the type of foods we could bring for lunch. The 1970s at Erieview Elementary School was definitely a different era. Today in most towns across the US, 50 percent of American children now suffer from chronic illnesses—more than at any other time in our history. Chronic childhood illnesses have gone from being a rarity to the norm.

- One in every eleven children has asthma in the US.[1]
- One in five has eczema (and it's on a steady increase in industrialized countries).[2]
- One out of four children experiences recurrent ear infections by age seven.[3]
- One in twelve has food allergies.[4]
- One in three has food sensitivities.

- One in eighty has celiac disease.[5]
- One in five is obese.[6]
- One in five has mental or behavioral impairments such as ADHD.[7]

In other words, we're sicker than we've ever been, and if our children are the future, the future is *not* healthy.

In this book, we'll explore children's health—especially chronic illness—through a new lens: through the eyes of an integrative pediatrician and an integrative pharmacist/mother of triplets. When you learn how to see and pay attention to the signs that your child's body is showing you, the path to healing is more clear and easier to follow.

> This book is loaded with case studies and a step-by-step guide to addressing chronic childhood illnesses using my HKHM program. With that said, this program is not appropriate for children who have severe food allergies; are underweight; have a G-tube; have severe pickiness or disordered eating; have a serious illness such as lupus, cystic fibrosis, chronic Lyme disease, or cancer; or have an undiagnosed illness.

GENETICS AND ILLNESS

Early in my career, while taking a family medical history, I listened for incidences of family illnesses to help discern whether the child's issue was an isolated case or could be due to genetics. Now I know how to look beyond genetics for further insights by identifying inflammation from food and other sources.

Here's a case from my own coffers. At the age of forty, I discovered I had a gluten sensitivity—as do one of my sisters, both of my parents, and one of my nieces. None of us meet the medical diagnostic criteria for celiac disease, but we all had health issues that either resolved completely or improved significantly when we stopped eating gluten. These included constipation, hemorrhoids, stomach pain, bloating, excess gas, weight gain, brain fog, joint pain, rosacea (red rash on the cheeks), anemia, and lack of energy. This certainly sounds like something with a genetic basis, doesn't it?

> Celiac disease is an autoimmune condition where the body reacts to gluten. Gluten is the protein found in wheat, barley, and rye. The disease can cause a host of different symptoms including gastrointestinal (GI) issues such as abdominal pain, constipation or loose stools, hemorrhoids, stomach pain, bloating, weight gain or weight loss, skin rashes, low energy, difficulty focusing (brain fog), or fatigue.

Dr. William Davis, a cardiologist who wrote the book *Wheat Belly*, would describe what my family members and I have as antibody-negative gluten sensitivity. We have many celiac disease symptoms, but our bodies don't make the classic antibody we test for in conventional laboratory tests. (We'll discuss testing in chapter 4.)

The discussion about gluten and my family always reminds me of my beloved paternal grandmother who we called Gram. She had stomach issues and ulcers her entire life and ended up dying with lymphoma. Individuals with undiagnosed celiac disease who continue to eat gluten have a three times higher rate of lymphoma than the general population.[8] The good news, however, is that once you go off gluten and your gut heals, your risk of lymphoma decreases to the same rate as that of the general population.[9] I now suspect that she may have had celiac disease, or possibly what the rest of us have, but she was just never diagnosed with it.

I will tell you more about my experience with gluten later, but the upshot is that a conventionally trained medical doctor with little nutrition training on the subtle differences among food allergies, food sensitivities, food intolerance, histamine intolerance, and celiac disease would likely have told me that I didn't need to be off gluten because I didn't have celiac disease or a true food allergy to wheat. If I'd started eating it again, my symptoms would have all come flooding back, and I would have ended up with a diagnosis of fibromyalgia or chronic fatigue syndrome.

My personal medical situation is part of what motivates my passion for identifying food sensitivities in children. It took me more than ten years to realize that the food I was eating was causing my GI issues. It took me that long, despite the many years of conventional *and* integrative medical training I had been through. The purpose of this book is to shorten the learning curve for you parents.

Now, back to my grandmother for a moment. Assessing a family medical history includes understanding ethnic tendencies toward certain diseases, which can also provide significant information. For instance, celiac disease is more prevalent in people of Northern European descent, specifically Irish, Scottish, and English. I have Irish, Scottish, and German roots, so I need to pay attention to my symptoms, my family's history, and my ethnic background. Sickle cell anemia is another good example: it is more prevalent in people of African, Central and South American, Middle Eastern, Asian, Indian, and Mediterranean descent.

Because of my personal experience and my integrative medical training, the way I interpret a child's history now is very different from the way I did fifteen years ago. Conventional medicine trains doctors to look for the diagnosis and treat it with medications and/or surgery. In integrative medicine, we are trained to look for patterns and view all symptoms as related, aiming to uncover the underlying cause of the inflammation. (We'll talk about this more in chapter 2.)

One system is not superior to the other—they simply have different perspectives and scopes. Each system has its place. Conventional medicine, better sanitation, and improved nutrition are the collective reasons our children are far more likely to live through childhood now than they were a hundred years ago. It's also the reason women typically survive childbirth and why we survive inflamed appendices, childhood kidney infections, and other formerly fatal ailments.

GENETICS AND EPIGENETICS

Looking through an integrative medical lens and taking into account an emerging field of research called *epigenetics*, we now know that our environment—including things such as food, environmental allergies, environmental toxins, infectious diseases, and stress—can influence our individual genetic expression.[10]

The old model told us that our genes are fixed and whatever diseases our parents or grandparents had, we will also likely have. For example, if your father died of a heart attack at forty-five, there's a good chance you will have a heart attack at forty-five. What epigenetics shows us is that certain things such as heart disease are not set in stone. Rather, it is the interaction of our DNA (genetic makeup) with all aspects of our environment that impacts our health. One good example is green leafy vegetables. Research has shown that a component of green leafy vegetables (methylators) can turn off genes that we don't necessarily want turned on.

The researchers took pregnant mice that were overweight, yellow, and diabetic. They fed them methylators during their pregnancy and the babies came out brown, normal weight, and non-diabetic.[11,12,13] I'll never forget when Chris Magryta, MD, my friend and a brilliant integrative pediatrician here in Charlotte, told me about this research. It's drop-your-jaw, fall-off-your-chair kind of info for us doctors. To be able to change the genetic expression of the offspring was just not heard of. Epigenetics gives us a *huge* bag of hope for all children. We can start where we are and make great headway.

> *Epi* means *above*, so epigenetics refers to the material above the genome that can cause activation and deactivation of genes, without a change in the underlying DNA.

When I review the family history, I highlight certain aspects to give parents an even more compelling reason to make nutritional changes that can have such a profound impact on their child's health.

family history of chemical dependency and addiction

Another crucial part of the family history pertains to chemical dependency and addiction. These often can lead an individual to self-medicate for some undiagnosed or untreated issue, such as anxiety, depression, ADD/ADHD, anger, learning issues, or chronic pain.

If a child is struggling in school or dealing with anger or anxiety, that child may be showing signs of a particularly important aspect of the family history. Is it possible that Grandpa, who was an alcoholic most of his life, actually had anxiety? Was alcohol the only way he knew how to manage?

If we explore the family history in this way, it helps us better understand our children. If we can recognize anxiety in a child at the age of seven versus twenty-seven, imagine all the tools with which we can equip that child. Even more, think about the stress, relationship dysfunction, miscommunications, and heartache we can potentially help her move through more gracefully, by identifying and treating her underlying anxiety.

Figuring out what health issues your family members may have struggled with can be the most challenging part of this process. Some families don't talk about health issues, especially those related to mental health. It also might be difficult to remember illnesses grandparents experienced.

I take epigenetics into account with every child I am seeing, even those with underlying genetic changes. For example, we know a child with Down syndrome has an extra copy of the twenty-first chromosome. This mutation is fixed and will result in certain cognitive and physical changes. For example, the anatomy of the ear canal, Eustachian tube, nasal passages, palate, and back of the mouth may be smaller than that of a child who does not have trisomy 21, putting them at higher risk for issues such as ear infections and sleep apnea. To solidify the concept of epigenetics, I'll share a case from my clinic.

Epigenetics taught me to look at children's illnesses and inflammation in the context of their environment and not assume simply because they may have different anatomy from other children that their inflammatory issues and illnesses are set in stone.

CASE STUDY

MARCUS

SYMPTOMS: EAR INFECTIONS, SINUS INFECTIONS, SLEEP APNEA, CONSTIPATION

Marcus's transformation blew my mind. His constellation of symptoms was extremely complicated, but his mother turned his health around just by listening to a talk I gave at our local children's library. After my presentation that day, she went home and made the changes I talked about. Six months later she brought nine-year-old Marcus to see me.

What she had done with his health was beyond impressive. Marcus's mother was another sign to me that I needed to compile this information into a book, so every interested parent could access it.

Marcus was a cute boy with Down syndrome and autism. I distinctly remembered his mother, because she'd asked great questions during the talk. I thought, *Wow—this mother gets it!* I share his case here because he is an example of one aspect of genetics that is fixed. He has an extra twenty-first chromosome, and green leafy vegetables will not change that; however, the constellation of inflammatory symptoms that he was struggling with can be shifted.

In the office, we reviewed his history. Marcus had nearly every one of the common childhood inflammatory illnesses that I am addressing in this book. Marcus had six sets of ear tubes for recurrent ear infections, surgery for recurrent sinus infections, and he had such bad sleep apnea that he had his tonsils and adenoids removed, and part of the base of his tongue was resected. (These procedures helped to open his airways, so he could get enough oxygen while sleeping.)

He also had severe constipation and eczema. His skin was very dry and rough, and he'd been on countless rounds of antibiotics.

After the library talk, Marcus's mother took him off dairy and gluten, started a probiotic, increased his omega-3 fats with fish oil, and started a vitamin D supplement. His lifelong constipation resolved fairly quickly, and his nasal congestion improved somewhat. However, even though the ear infections slowed, he was still requiring antibiotics every three to four months.

His mother and I decided to do some IgG food sensitivity testing on him. (I'll discuss this more in depth in chapter 4.) I don't order this test often because it doesn't have strong scientific reliability. In situations like Marcus's, I find it helpful when we interpret the test results in the context of his overall clinical picture and keep its limitations in mind.

His test results were positive for many foods, including gluten and dairy. Mom felt confident she could remove the additional foods from his diet, and since she loved to cook, she proceeded to shift his diet yet again, while keeping him off gluten and dairy.

Normally, we remove these foods for three to six months and then add them back. However, Marcus was doing so well with these foods out of his diet that she kept his IgG-positive foods out of his diet for an entire year. She also decided to take all grains out of his diet.

One year after being on this anti-inflammatory diet, she exclaimed, "He's never been better!" It was the first time in his life that he went an entire year without a single antibiotic.

He did continue to experience some mild nasal congestion, but his parents controlled it with a saltwater nasal rinse using a neti pot. Marcus's mother taught him how to do the rinse himself.

He was still on the autism spectrum, but he was significantly less hyperactive and less aggressive. (Previously, they'd tried a stimulant medication for the hyperactivity, but it didn't help.) Furthermore, the ear tube fell out of his right ear (the one from his sixth set), and his ENT doctor thought for sure Marcus's ear infections would return. They never did.

Marcus is a testament to the power of nutrition. Changing your child's diet can be a tremendous amount of work, but the effort is worth it in the end. Once the child's systemic inflammation has decreased and his system is back in balance, you typically don't have to be as strict with the diet. But that depends on the child and how sensitive his body is.

Our conventional medical system trained me to look at Marcus in parts. Sleep apnea is separate from constipation, which is separate from recurrent ear infections, eczema, and hyperactivity. Integrative medicine taught me that all of these are related and worsened by inflammation, and once we figured out the inflammatory triggers, we could begin to decrease that overall body inflammation.

As we decreased Marcus's excessive systemic inflammation, some of his chronic congestion and mucus buildup improved. This allowed his Eustachian tubes to drain more effectively, potentially lessening his recurrent ear infections. Air could also pass through his nasal passages more easily, possibly lessening recurrent sinus infections. His gut inflammation lessened, improving his constipation and eczema, and with less inflammation and better nutrient absorption, his immune system could start functioning more efficiently, so he did not end up on antibiotics once a month.

As you can see from Marcus's story, this transformation doesn't happen overnight. We slowly and methodically work to rebalance the overriding inflammation in these kids. That's what we'll explore in the following chapters.

TAKEAWAYS

- Integrative medicine is a powerful combination of conventional medicine partnered with natural and nutritional therapies. The blend of both systems taps into the body's innate healing capabilities.
- One in two children today suffers from a chronic illness.
- Epigenetics is an emerging field of research outlining the way our genes interact with the environment. Nutrition is a powerful tool to optimize gene expression and overall health.
- Armed with the right information, guidance, and structure, the nutrition and supplement recommendations I make in section II of the book offer the possibility of changing your child's health forever.

CHAPTER 2

to understand illness, first understand inflammation

MARCUS'S STORY IN CHAPTER 1 is a profound case for understanding the role that genes, nutrition, our environment, and epigenetics plays in our overall health. We removed certain foods as a part of an anti-inflammatory diet for Marcus and saw profound improvements in his many inflammatory conditions (eczema, recurrent ear and sinus infections, constipation, and hyperactivity). But before we go any further, we need to have a shared understanding of what I mean by inflammation and its role in our health.

When most of us think of inflammation, we see images of a hot, puffy, red, irritated, and painful body part, like when a cut gets infected. However, inflammation is more than an acute response to injury, and it's not always just localized to one part of our body. Inflammation is an intricate, complex response by the whole body to what it perceives as a threat.

This means the body can have an inflammatory response for many reasons—not just from infection but also from irritants, allergies (food and environmental), and even stress. If we think of inflammation as the body's self-protection mode, we can understand how and why inflammation can become chronic and spread throughout the body.

To some extent, we need inflammation. If we cut a finger, we need the inflammatory process in that area to stop the bleeding. If we sprain an ankle, we need white blood cells to go to that area and begin to repair the damaged tissues. But when inflammation goes unchecked, and the body keeps mounting an inflammatory response to the same trigger, it leads to chronic inflammation and disease. Integrative medicine teaches us that we need to look not only at *why* the body is responding to a trigger but also at *what* that trigger is.

A HELPFUL INFLAMMATION ANALOGY

Think of a glass of water. The glass is the body, and the water is the inflammation in the body. Our bodies have a baseline level of inflammation, depending upon the five contributing factors to inflammation (genetics plus food, environmental allergies, environmental toxins, infectious diseases, and stress, both emotional and physical), which I'll talk about shortly.

Excess inflammation leads to worsening symptoms. When we minimize inflammation, we minimize symptoms.

INFLAMMATION AND ILLNESS

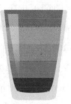

Chronic excess
Inflammation

Well-controlled
inflammation

Let's look at a specific example, an eight-year-old girl named Sara. Sara has eczema, asthma, allergies, chronic runny nose, and constipation; eats the standard American diet (SAD) of processed foods (high sugar content and artificial dyes); has environmental allergies to trees and grasses; and lives in an area with high levels of air pollution. You can see in the image below that she has a significant amount of systemic inflammation and her glass of water is overflowing, which prevents her immune system from working effectively and efficiently.

Since we can't cut down all the trees and dig up all the grasses, we look at the aspect of Sara's environment that we have the most control over: food. We minimize her processed and packaged foods; add in more vegetables, healthy fats, and proteins; replace high-sugar drinks with water; and remove dairy from her diet.

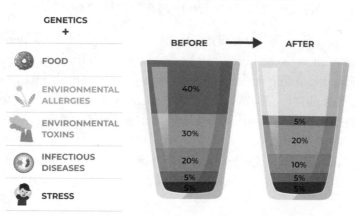

SARA'S CUP OF INFLAMMATION

GENETICS +

FOOD

ENVIRONMENTAL ALLERGIES

ENVIRONMENTAL TOXINS

INFECTIOUS DISEASES

STRESS

BEFORE → AFTER

40% / 5%

30% / 20%

20% / 10%

5% / 5%

5% / 5%

As we begin to decrease systemic inflammation, the glass will go from overflowing down to half-full or less. Sara's cellular health improves. This somewhat decreases the impact the air pollution and environmental allergies have on her body. When spring and fall allergy seasons come along, or Sara is exposed to more pollution or a virus, her inflammation goes up and her glass starts to fill, but now it's only three-fourths full. For a change, she may get through allergy season with little to no allergy medication and she may not need her albuterol rescue inhaler as much as she did the previous seasons. Possibly even the MiraLAX she's been taking for two years for constipation is no longer needed.

The higher the amount of baseline inflammation, the longer it may take to get the inflammation under control. Sometimes this means adding more medications or supplements at first to treat the child's illness and to strengthen her immune system.

Sounds simple, right?

The concept of inflammation and illness *is* simple, but the body and all of its moving parts are complex. We also have to consider all the other aspects of a child's environment in order to bring her inflammation to a minimum.

INFLAMMATION:
Three Major Concepts

I'd like to introduce you to three major concepts regarding inflammation, which I wish I'd learned in medical school. In the next several pages, I'll teach you what it took me over fifteen years to learn!

1. Most physical symptoms of illnesses stem from inflammation.
2. Physical signs and symptoms of inflammation are often related.
3. Five things trigger inflammation in our bodies.
   Food
   Environmental allergies
   Environmental toxins
   Infectious diseases
   Stress

It is the interaction of our genes with these triggers that determines our overall health. Our bodies don't have fences. Inflammatory cells can travel anywhere in the body, from the gut to the brain to the skin. Therefore, poorly controlled asthma *is* related to constipation and stomachaches. Recurrent ear infections *are* related to uncontrolled eczema. This also applies to our central nervous system. Have you ever noticed that your child's behavior is worse if he has gone three or four days without a bowel moment? Or at the height of allergy season, does he seem more irritable? If a child has tics, I often see them worsen during allergy season.

MAJOR CONCEPT 1:
Most Physical Symptoms of Illness
Stem from Inflammation

By now, you are familiar with the list of inflammatory illnesses in kids: reflux, eczema, keratosis pilaris (bumps on the back of the arms), recurrent ear or sinus infections, chronic runny nose, allergies, asthma, stomach pain, and constipation or loose stools.

Some signs of these illnesses may be more obvious than others. We can easily see the skin and the inside of the nose, but it's harder to get a clear picture of what's going on inside the body. Acne and eczema are easy to see, whereas the cause for wheezing takes a little more work to discover because the inflammation is deeper and not visible to the unaided eye.

The prevalence of coexisting conditions is why I always talk about the "constellation of symptoms." Some of the more obvious signs of inflammation can guide us into understanding the deeper inflammation that might be happening with your child. The subtler, more "silent" types of inflammation can fester undetected for years, which can also cause consequences later in life.

An example of this silent inflammatory process in adults is heart disease. Doctors now know that heart disease (more accurately termed cardiovascular disease) is related to chronic inflammation, which causes plaque buildup in arteries. It takes years to build up enough plaque to obstruct arteries, but when an artery that supplies blood to the heart is finally blocked, it can no longer supply enough blood and oxygen to the heart muscle, leading to a heart attack.

The underlying signs of inflammation may not be obvious either until it's too late, as with a heart attack or stroke (which is the same process as with the heart, but instead the vessels are blocked in the brain), or until it has been building up for years, damaging the tissues and hindering the ability of the heart to pump blood effectively.

Another disease that can provide insight about underlying inflammation is asthma. Asthma can seem elusive and below the surface if you don't understand how pervasive and irritating the inflammatory cells are to the lungs in an individual who wheezes. Patients with asthma often have many more visible signs of inflammation, such as eczema, bumps on the backs of the arms (keratosis pilaris), dark circles under the eyes, chronic nasal congestion, runny nose, and constipation.

Please bear with me here even if your child doesn't have asthma. This discussion provides some important information that will give you a broader understanding of inflammation, disease, and health.

Asthma is characterized by excess inflammation in the body, the lungs in particular. When a child with asthma is exposed to one of her "asthma triggers," such as tree pollen, tobacco smoke, or even a virus, her immune system says, "Hello, invader! Let me send an army of cells to the lungs, so I can get rid of you!"

The body then sends a whoosh of white blood cells (mucus) to the lungs. The mucus irritates the muscles in the airways and causes them to constrict. This constriction is what leads to wheezing. It's a complex dance among allergies, the immune system, genetics, and inflammation, as we'll see in Gary's case. As you read it, you'll notice the five triggers of inflammation.

CASE STUDY

GARY

SYMPTOM: RECURRENT WHEEZING

Gary was four years old when his mother brought him to see me. He'd had a persistent cough for several months. Throughout the previous two years, he'd had recurrent bouts of coughing, runny nose, and wheezing that required an albuterol inhaler. For the wheezing, he'd taken one course of oral steroids, which he did not tolerate. His behavior became erratic, with irritability, mood swings, and sleep troubles.

At that point, his mother knew she never wanted him to take oral steroids again. She decided to switch to an integrative pediatrician. She felt the conventional medical approach was aimed at treating his symptoms, and her intuition was telling her his chronic cough and congestion had some underlying cause that wasn't being addressed.

Gary's mother and I combed through his history. As an infant, he had been extremely fussy and colicky and later developed recurrent bouts of wheezing, coughing, and chronic nasal congestion. During his office visit, I observed that he was a mouth breather; he had a runny nose and dark, puffy circles under his eyes; and his breathing was audible (which I affectionately call "Darth Vader breathing"). All of these signs indicated uncontrolled systemic inflammation.

On exam, the inside of his nose (nasal mucosa) was pale in color, almost bluish, and swollen shut, which made him a mouth breather.

Environmental allergies often cause the nasal mucosa to be pale and swollen. As luck would have it, Gary's previous pediatrician had done allergy testing through bloodwork and discovered a severe dust mite allergy. My first question when a child has a dust mite allergy is: How old are his mattress and pillows?

Mattresses and pillows are dust mite havens. One study, conducted at a London hospital, suggested that up to a third of a pillow's weight could be made up of bugs, dead skin, and dust mites and their feces.

Gary happened to be sleeping on a fifteen-year-old mattress from his uncle's college days. Given the severity of his dust mite allergy, his mother and I decided they should invest in a new mattress and pillows. Then they could put plastic covers over them to prevent dust mites from settling into them. These covers would help us keep Gary's dust mite exposure to a minimum while he slept.

MAJOR CONCEPT 2:
Physical Signs and Symptoms Are All Related to One Another

Our traditional medical system has moved toward treating symptoms, and looking at the body, in a reductionist fashion. A person will see a dermatologist to prescribe steroids for eczema, an ENT doctor for ear tubes, and then a gastroenterologist for a laxative prescription for constipation. This routine is typical for many of my patients.

Often, doctors are treating *symptoms* of illness instead of figuring out the *root* of the illness. And while it may sound as if I'm pointing a critical finger at conventional medicine, I'm not. As I've previously stated, conventional and integrative medicine are equally important. But I'm saying that we physicians must take a step back and look at our training. Doctors are trained to find exactly where a tumor is and how to either remove it with surgery or shrink it with chemotherapy. A great deal of research money goes toward treatments. However, we need more research on what may have triggered the tumor growth in the first place and what type of nutrition and lifestyle modifications might help support the patient's body to get through the treatment more smoothly and possibly prevent it from reoccurring.

I liken my job as a physician to that of a car mechanic. I need to look beneath the hood and, when possible, remove or resolve whatever is causing the symptoms. If my car had a recurrent issue—let's say the headlights kept going out—I'd take it to a mechanic. If he fixed it and two weeks later the lights went out again, I'd take the car to a different mechanic, perhaps one who specializes in the electrical circuitry of cars. This mechanic will get in there, figure out where the wiring is off, and fix it, while helping me understand the bigger picture of the problem. I'd continue to go to my original mechanic for oil changes and other maintenance, but if I have a more complex or recurring problem, I might go to a mechanic who has more time, a different toolbox, and more diagnostic equipment.

Most physicians prefer to figure out the underlying cause of an illness, including me. In conventional medicine, however, we often have little time with patients. My medical training emphasized the "allergy march." This refers to the natural history or typical progression of allergic diseases that often begin early in life and include atopic dermatitis (eczema), food allergy, allergic rhinitis (runny nose due to allergies), and asthma. My tools for controlling symptoms at that time were antihistamines and steroids. At that time, I didn't understand about cumulative inflammation and its five triggers. Of the five, I knew the least about how inflammatory foods could, in some cases, worsen allergy symptoms.

Many of you have been reading about nutrition, researching supplements, and asking your pediatricians for advice. Before I did my integrative medical training, bringing your child to me and asking nutrition and supplement advice was like taking your electric car to a diesel mechanic. Both mechanics know engines, but the tools they use are somewhat different. I simply didn't have enough (or any) nutrition training to really give any advice. But I also didn't know nutrition could even be playing a role. I just knew I needed to ask whether the child was eating vegetables and drinking two to three cups of milk per day.

When I was first out of residency, I used medications to treat the symptoms of the allergy march with patients like Gary. I would have prescribed an inhaled steroid for him, along with an antihistamine for allergies, a topical steroid for the eczema, and a nasal steroid spray for his runny nose. This would have addressed most of his inflammatory symptoms during the time of year when his allergies and asthma flared up the most. If he had constipation on top of all that, I would have also given him a laxative.

When I know a child has an increased risk of asthma or any other type of inflammatory issue like allergies, constipation, or reflux, I now look at the bigger picture and ask, *How can I reduce this child's overall systemic inflammation?*

I then utilize the system I've developed based upon my integrative medical training and years of experience in pinpointing what may be triggering a child's wheezing—the very system you're learning about in this book.

MAJOR CONCEPT 3:
Five Things Trigger Inflammation in Our Bodies

Keep in mind that we all have differences in our underlying genetics that impact the way we respond to everything in our environment, from foods to viruses to stress. Think about the five triggers as anything in our environment that our bodies can react to.

Let's go back to Gary's case. For kids who wheeze at a young age, we stratify them into risk categories: those who will likely go on to develop asthma and those who will just wheeze until they are about two or three years old with colds, but then they will outgrow it. Given Gary's symptoms, as well as his family history of asthma, he was in the highest risk category and was almost ten times more likely to develop persistent asthma.[1]

Gary's signs of inflammation can be classic for someone with a dairy sensitivity and also for an environmental allergen such as dust mites. We identified ways we could decrease his systemic inflammation—to get his wheezing, runny nose, and cough under control—starting with two of the five areas of inflammation: food and environmental allergies.

TRIGGER	HOW WE DIAGNOSED	HOW WE TREATED
Food	My professional experience indicated that dairy was most likely contributing to his overall systemic inflammation.	We eliminated dairy, since he had a classic history of a cow-milk protein sensitivity, which caused colic, reflux, and a chronic runny nose. We also added some key supplements including probiotics, vitamin D, fish oil, magnesium, and a whole food supplement.
Environmental Allergies	An IgE Environmental Allergy Profile was done through bloodwork. This can also be done by an allergist with skin prick testing.	He had a severe dust mite allergy, so his parents got rid of the old mattress and pillows he was sleeping on.

TRIGGER	HOW WE DIAGNOSED	HOW WE TREATED
Environmental Toxins	Nothing in his medical history made me suspicious of an environmental toxin; therefore, we did not test.	We didn't need to address anything in this category with him.
Infectious Diseases	I diagnosed Gary with walking pneumonia at his first visit by listening to his lungs. We treated this with an antibiotic. If I had suspected a more serious type of pneumonia, I would have referred him for a chest x-ray.	Gary's wheezing episodes were triggered by two main things: his allergies (dust mites) and viruses (infectious microorganisms). Once we removed inflammatory triggers like milk and dust mites, his systemic inflammation decreased, and his immune system became more efficient and effective at fighting off viruses and bacteria.
Stress	Lack of sleep increases stress to the child's system and holds them in the sick cycle because it dampens their immune function. In Gary's case, his sleep deprivation also manifested in behavioral issues. So, while Gary wasn't sleeping, neither were his parents, and everyone's glass of stress was overflowing!	We shifted Gary out of crisis mode, which lifted him out of the sick cycle and significantly decreased his and his parents' stress level.

At his follow-up appointment three weeks later, Gary's chronic nasal congestion and cough had almost completely resolved. Eventually, the dark circles under his eyes disappeared, as did his mouth breathing. His need for albuterol decreased.

FIVE TRIGGERS OF INFLAMMATION

GENETICS
+

FOOD
Processed, packaged foods, artificial dyes and colors, refined sugar

Food allergies, food sensitivities, celiac disease, food intolerance, and histamine intolerance

ENVIRONMENTAL ALLERGIES

Indoor allergens
cats, dogs, dust mites, mold, insects including cockroaches

Outdoor allergens
pollen (grass, trees, weeds), mold

ENVIRONMENTAL TOXINS

Mold toxins
found in water-damaged buildings

Heavy metals or chemicals
herbicides (glyphosate) or pesticides

INFECTIOUS DISEASES
Bacteria
Viruses
Fungi
Parasites
Protozoans
Prions

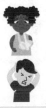

PHYSICAL STRESS
Broken bone, herniated disc, torticollis (tight neck muscle in babies), Eustachian tube dysfunction

EMOTIONAL STRESS
Relationships, abuse, family dynamics, cultural expectations, jobs, negative self talk, guilt

GARY'S CUP OF INFLAMMATION

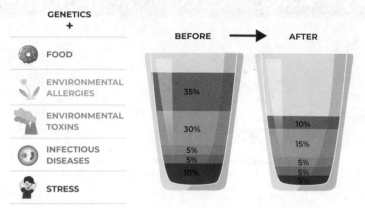

Gary improved rapidly, and to this day, he is doing great. He is one of hundreds of children whom I have seen over the years who have enjoyed an improved path with their wheezing or asthma after we methodically worked to decrease their systemic inflammation.

I've heard this question many times from parents: why didn't anybody tell us that food could be contributing to the illness? My response is always the same: when I trained, nutrition wasn't part of the curriculum. If I'd seen your child before I started studying nutrition and integrative medicine, I would've given you the same advice your previous pediatrician gave you.

Gary's situation was straightforward. The dark circles under his eyes and his Darth Vader breathing are easy to identify in kids and adults when you know what you are looking for. But some cases are more complex and require further probing. One of my goals with this book is to help you see and identify the inflammation in your child, so it can be resolved sooner.

TAKEAWAYS

- Life is made up of a set of complex variables impacting us at all times, including illness. By breaking down the main triggers of inflammation into an easily understood, organized fashion, you can begin to understand how to gain control of your child's health.
- The important thing is to be pragmatic and remember that each trigger of inflammation carries equal weight. If we address one area with 100 percent effort but ignore the others, you may not see the true health transformation you're seeking for your child.
- Understanding these triggers of inflammation can also help you to partner more easily with your child's doctor to find the root of illness more efficiently.

CHAPTER 3

leaky gut vs. healthy gut

I LIVED IN A HOUSE with ten girls in college. Somebody was always waiting for me to get out of the bathroom. My constipation was ever-present. Each time I needed to move my bowels, it felt like child-birth. And it was always touch-and-go whether or not it would happen. Wow, I cannot believe I am writing this—if you see me around town with a bag on my head, you'll know why.

I also had stomach discomfort almost every time I ate, but just thought that was how everyone felt after eating. I didn't know any different. On top of that, I was diagnosed with an autoimmune condition, Hashimoto's hypothyroidism, as I was starting medical school. I had no idea at the time that food could be playing a role in my consti-pation, abdominal discomfort, or thyroid issue.

Fast forward to my integrative medical training, and I began under-standing nutrition and health. I started advising parents how to deal with constipated children by removing dairy from their diets, but somehow, I still wasn't connecting the dots in my own life. I had a bowel movement every day, so I didn't think my bowels and the time and effort it took to go were even a *thing*.

I was taking patients off gluten and dairy and seeing magic happen. Bowels were beginning to function properly, lifelong stomachaches were going away, the allergy march diseases were improving (eczema, allergies, asthma), and, as an added bonus, behavior, focus, and sleep were improving. Parents were noticing fewer meltdowns, outbursts, and mood swings.

Around this time, my sister (who also has hypothyroidism) took gluten out of her diet and felt a whole lot better. I decided to take the plunge. It was remarkable, as if someone took a bag off my head. Suddenly (within days), I had a clear head, I had no energy slumps after eating, and my bowel movements were so much easier (but they still took a little while). In addition, my stomach stopped hurting after every meal, and my skin took on a new glow. I had been through all of this schooling and training—four years of traditional medical school, three years of pediatric residency, two years of integrative medical fellowship—in addition to five or six years of clinical practice, and I was just *now* figuring out I had a food sensitivity much of my life?

I actually think my constipation started in college. I don't remember having bowel issues or recurrent abdominal pain in childhood. When I think back to my cup of college inflammation, I had a significant increase in gluten, dairy, and processed foods (that my mother did not keep in our house), in addition to increased stress and lack of exercise (a big stress reliever for me). My cup was overflowing.

SHEILA'S CUP OF INFLAMMATION

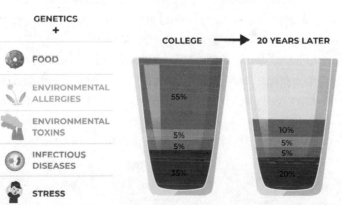

The longer I remained off gluten, the better I felt. It made me realize that I had previously become one of those people who eats because I had to eat, not because I enjoyed food.

About a year after I went off gluten, I attended a medical conference where one of the speakers said, "Bowel movements should only take you the same amount of time it takes you to urinate."

Wait, what?!

She was discussing the role of nutrition and how it impacts the gut—no pun intended! In particular, she was extolling the virtues of a gluten-free, dairy-free diet for some people.

The concept that moving your bowels should be quick, easy, and without strain did not even compute with me. But this doctor had said it, and it made sense when I thought back to what I knew about the physiology of our GI system. As I listened to this lecture on bowel movements and thought about the notion that they *should* be quick *and easy*, I thought once again about the connection between my bowels and my diet. *Should I also be off dairy?* I'd adjusted to losing one delicious food group in removing gluten. Was I prepared to lose another?

Dairy was a different story than gluten for me. Cheese was one of my favorite foods, and as a busy pediatrician, cheese was easy. There was no cooking or preparing; I could just grab a slice on the go and feel satiated for another couple of hours.

Nonetheless, I decided to give it up. Although my bowel movements had gotten tremendously easier since I had gone off gluten, when I went off dairy as well, I could get in and out of the bathroom with the speed and efficiency of a NASCAR pit crew. The disco ball dropped out of the ceiling again, and I had my own private dance party.

 Disco ball - my AHA moment!

I really didn't know bowel movements could be so easy. And then I was in for another surprise six months after I went off dairy. I did a brief cleanse with a like-minded group. For three weeks we took gluten, dairy, sugar, all animal products, caffeine, and alcohol out of our diets. From a bowel movement perspective, doing this cleanse was like heaven, and I felt fantastic. However, I couldn't keep up that level of elimination for much longer than three weeks, but it served an essential purpose: It showed me how my body could function and helped me establish a different baseline of eating. It also gave me great insight into how I could further help my patients and their parents understand what was going on.

What I have learned from my practice and from my own health is that bowel rhythms give us a window into inflammation and gut health. From an integrative medicine perspective, the gut is the body's powerhouse—the system that can set the tone for the body's other systems.

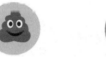

I have remained off gluten and dairy for many years, but over the past couple of years I have been able to loosen up the reins on dairy. I eat Kerrygold grass-fed butter almost daily, and occasionally I will have regular cheese on a gluten-free pizza. I can do that now because I gave my gut time to heal. My GI system, skin, energy, and ability to think clearly after eating a meal have remained significantly better than when I was eating a lot of gluten and dairy on a daily basis.

Not everyone has an issue with gluten and dairy, which is why I recommend doing a selective elimination diet to test out the waters. They are both yummy foods and if your child's system can handle them, there is no need for her to be strictly off of them. The best way to find out is to remove them one at a time (as we do in the program) and monitor symptoms to see if there is a change. For me, gluten is more problematic than dairy and I find it is often the case that one or the other makes more of a difference with many kids as well.

THE SCOOP ON POOP

My first and highest priority when working with a child is to get her gut in order. We want daily, easy, formed stools. Review the Bristol stool chart I have included for handy visualization. It categorizes stool quality; the goal is a 3 or 4—like a sausage or a snake—I know, gross. Stools should be quick and should not not be a major, foul-smelling event. They will be stinky, yes, but not clear-the-room foul. Daily easy stools are one of our first indictors of a healthy gut.

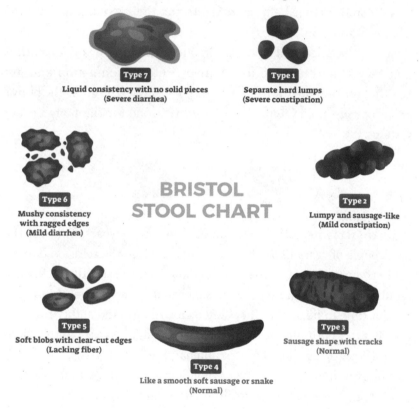

BRISTOL STOOL CHART

Type 7
Liquid consistency with no solid pieces
(Severe diarrhea)

Type 1
Separate hard lumps
(Severe constipation)

Type 6
Mushy consistency
with ragged edges
(Mild diarrhea)

Type 2
Lumpy and sausage-like
(Mild constipation)

Type 5
Soft blobs with clear-cut edges
(Lacking fiber)

Type 3
Sausage shape with cracks
(Normal)

Type 4
Like a smooth soft sausage or snake
(Normal)

What do we mean by the gut, exactly? The entire length of the GI tract—everything from the esophagus to the stomach to the small intestine, colon, and rectum—and the activity that begins the moment food is placed into the mouth and continues until it hits the toilet, constitutes the gut.

The gut is the hub for about 70 percent of our immune system. This might surprise you until you consider that it regulates the breakdown and absorption of food, it is often where skin issues stem from, and of course it governs our waste removal and detoxification.

A well-functioning GI system does more to keep the immune system—and the body itself—in balance than any supplement or medication could ever hope to. Fermented foods, fiber, and nutrients from our food, as well as being outside in nature and playing in the dirt, contribute significantly to the health of our GI tract. Together they enhance the content and diversity of the bacteria in the gut (also called the microbiome). This sets the stage for a strong, well-functioning, well-balanced immune system. We will discuss the microbiome in more detail later in this chapter.

LEAKY GUT
(INCREASED INTESTINAL PERMEABILITY)

A connection exists among the environment of the gut, inflammation, environmental allergies, food allergies, food sensitivities, and autoimmune diseases (recall my diagnosis of Hashimoto's hypothyroidism) that I didn't learn about during medical school and residency. Here's how it works.

We have a single layer of cells along our GI tract, and the health and integrity of this layer of cells, called our *epithelial cell layer,* is critical for our overall health and immune system. Each cell is cemented to another by something called a *tight junction.* When these tight junctions begin to break down, the medical term is *increased intestinal permeability.* But most people have come to call it "leaky gut," which describes an unhealthy gut lining and gut environment.

If we expose our gut and microbiome to certain foods (artificial dyes, processed foods, refined sugar), medications (antacids, unnecessary antibiotics, steroids), or environmental toxins (herbicides or pesticides), this interferes with the growth of *beneficial* bacteria in the gut and also creates inflammation. This inflammation damages the epithelial cells and the tight junctions, making the gut more permeable. The body then begins to absorb things into the bloodstream that shouldn't be there. Once these runaway molecules from the gut hit the bloodstream, they set off a cascade of inflammation because the body treats them as invaders.

When the gut is inflamed, our bodies struggle to effectively and efficiently absorb all the nutrients from our food. If this inflammation goes unchecked, it leads to nutrient deficiencies such as low iron, and it also spreads to many different systems. This inflamed or leaky gut lining is part of the reason children who have asthma also have eczema, bumps on the backs of their arms and cheeks, chronic runny nose, constipation, recurrent ear infections, and sometimes lots of meltdowns.[1] In conventional medicine, we look at all of these symptoms as separate illnesses, but in integrative medicine, we look at them as chronic, unchecked, systemic inflammation.

INFLAMMATION IN THE GUT IS INFLAMMATION EVERYWHERE

We don't have fences in the body, so when we have a leaky gut and undigested food particles are triggering a cascade of inflammation into our bloodstream, all our other systems can be affected, including our brain and nervous system.

For example, children who have constipation often have behavior and mood problems when they get to day two, three, or four of not having a bowel movement. The buildup of metabolic by-products resulting from poor digestion and excess inflammation can contribute to behavior issues. This can look like meltdowns in the younger kids and mood swings or emotional outbursts in older kids. The next time you start to discipline your constipated child, pause and look at the last time they pooped. See if you can get their bowels back on track with the HKHM program. Lean toward improving their digestive function and let's see if we can restore some semblance of harmony in your home!

The graphic "Healthy Gut vs. Leaky Gut" is a great illustration of how an unhealthy or leaky cell leads to a leaky gut, which leads to inflammation affecting the brain and central nervous system. When I first started using the selective elimination diet in my patients, we kept seeing these added perks of improved nutrition and digestion. The kids were sleeping better and more restfully, their meltdowns or mood swings improved, and some kids were able to focus better.

INFLAMMATION-LEAKY GUT-ILLNESSES

Circle the symptoms that apply to your child.

An unhealthy diet creates a leaky gut, causing inflammation and illness.

A healthy diet and supplements create a healthy gut, keeping our mind and body in balance.

- Headaches, trouble focusing
- Sleep disturbance, snoring, fatigue
- Mouth breathing, meltdowns
- Allergies, nasal congestion
- Recurrent ear and sinus infections

- Consistent full night's sleep
- Good focus and energy
- Clear breathing through the nose

- Asthma and wheezing
- Skin issues (eczema, bumps)

- Hydrated, healthy skin

- Bloating, gas, abdominal pain
- Food intolerances, weight gain

- Healthy gut, optimal nutrient absorption

- Constipation or loose stools
- Bright red ring around the anus

- Regular bowel movements

- Muscle cramps
- Early fatigue when playing
- Restless leg syndrome, "all over the bed"

- Muscles working well, able to keep up with other kids while playing

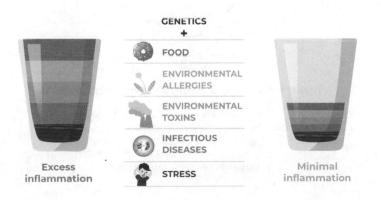

GENETICS
+

FOOD

ENVIRONMENTAL ALLERGIES

ENVIRONMENTAL TOXINS

INFECTIOUS DISEASES

STRESS

Excess inflammation

Minimal inflammation

HEALTHY GUT VS. LEAKY GUT

Leaky Gut

Unhealthy Gut Cell
Poor cell wall integrity, nutrient exchange, and cell signaling.
An unhealthy cell leads to unhealthy systems.

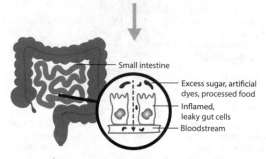

Leaky Gut Cells of the Small Intestine
Poorly digested food creates inflammation and damages the tight junctions.
This creates leakiness between cells, allowing toxins and undigested food
particles to access the bloodstream, which leads to inflammation.

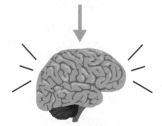

Brain & Nervous System Downstream Effects

- Emotional outbursts, frequent "meltdowns"
- Sleep issues (trouble falling asleep, staying asleep, restless leg)
- Fatigue
- Lack of focus
- Worsening behavior with constipation

HEALTHY GUT VS. LEAKY GUT

Healthy Gut

Gut Cell
Healthy cell with good fats making up the cell wall. Nutrients and cell signals are able to flow in and out of the cell easily.

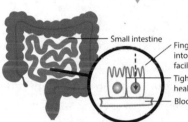

Small intestine

Finger-like projections extend into the small intestine and facilitate food absorption

Tight junctions between healthy cells

Bloodstream

Small Intestine
Nutrients absorbed effectively and efficiently. Inflammation is minimized with healthy digestion.

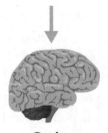

Brain
Efficient breakdown and absorption of fats and proteins help to support brain function, energy, and the ability to remain calm, focus, fall asleep, stay asleep, and much more.

Concept creation in conjunction with Deborah Allen, RPh, as an adaptation from the book *Leaky Cells, Leaky Gut, Leaky Brain*, with permission from the authors, Jess Armine, DC, and Elizma Lambert, ND.

Our world today is much more sterile than it was even twenty years ago—in some ways that is good. We die far less often from infectious diseases (except unfortunately during a pandemic), but our chronic diseases have skyrocketed. Could that in part be due to our increasingly sterile lives? Strong cleaning products, along with antibacterial soaps and hand sanitizers, are in widespread use. According to the FDA, exposure to triclosan, an ingredient in hand sanitizers that was banned in 2017 (as were twenty-three other ingredients), possibly contributed to making bacteria more resistant to antibiotics. It also poses other health risks, including thyroid hormone disruption and skin cancer. (See https://www.fda.gov/consumers/consumer-updates/5-things-know-about-triclosan.)

Hand sanitizers remain ever-present. Yes, it's important to keep our hands clean, but soap and water may be the best option for killing harmful bacteria and viruses, while maintaining the integrity of our skin and not creating bacterial super-strains that become resistant to antibiotics.

THE MICROBIOME

You know by now that the gut microbiome is the teeming ecosystem along the GI tract made up of bacteria, yeast, and other microorganisms that play a critical role in your child's overall health. Keeping these microscopic creatures alive and well fed is important to our overall health, although we did not learn about this in medical school.

This ecosystem is highly dependent on how we live our lives, what we eat, and what we are exposed to (our environment, stressors, medications). Take two children, one with a diverse and beneficial microbiome, the other with an unhealthy one. Expose them to the same classroom environment. One child might get the sniffles for a couple of days, but not miss a single day of school. The other might get sick and be out for a week every other month, often on rounds of antibiotics.

An analogy to gardening makes this easy to understand. A gardener wants nutrient-rich soil and uses clean water to encourage green, healthy plants to grow and thrive. A healthy gut microbiome helps us bounce back more quickly after being exposed to a virus or bacteria, just like a healthy plant can withstand an occasional dry spell.

GUT HEALTH

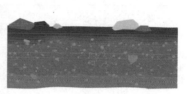

Healthy soil represents healthy gut microbiome

Depleted, dry soil represents unhealthy gut microbiome

FACTORS THAT MAY IMPACT OUR MICROBIOME

- Poor-quality processed food.
- Hand sanitizers and strong cleaning agents with bleach.[2] Living in such a sterile environment may actually be impacting the diversity of bacteria in our gut and therefore our overall health (referred to as the hygiene hypothesis).[3]
- Herbicides (containing glyphosate) that kill weeds and microorganisms in the soil. Widespread global use of glyphosate has increased dramatically since 1996 (fifteenfold).[4] It is used by the farming industry on crops and for nonagricultural use such private yards and schools.
- Antibiotics that kill bacteria causing an infection but also kill the beneficial bacteria in the gut. There were 270 million antibiotic prescriptions written in 2015; this is equivalent to about 838 antibiotic prescriptions for every 1,000 people.[5]
- Antibiotics used in food-producing animals have contributed significantly to resistant bacterial strains that impact human

health (3,500,000 kg of tetracycline was used in 2017, predominantly in the cattle and swine industries).[6]

- The high C-section rate in the US (up to 30 percent in some areas, a 60 percent increase from 1996 to 2011).[7] A C-section baby enters the world through a sterile surgical incision and does not descend through the birth canal. Therefore, the baby does not ingest the beneficial *Lactobacillus* bacteria from the wall of the vagina.

research on leaky gut and celiac disease

This groundbreaking concept of leaky gut has been understood by naturopathic doctors for years. It has only been more recently introduced to the conventional medical world by Alessio Fasano, MD, an Italian physician at Harvard, who is the head of pediatric gastroenterology and nutrition. His research has shown that patients with celiac disease (an autoimmune condition where gluten attacks the lining of the gut, causing damage) have higher levels of a molecule called *zonulin*. Zonulin damages the tight junctions between the cells that line the gut.[8]

Dr. Fasano's research also found that gluten triggered the zonulin elevation even in individuals who don't have celiac disease.[9] Some of you reading this book may have experienced this. I certainly have. My celiac test results through bloodwork are completely negative. I did not have an endoscopy since the bloodwork was negative and my symptoms all went away quickly and easily when I went off of gluten. I note this here because so many kids I see have a gluten sensitivity, but they don't have celiac disease. I test kids before taking them off of gluten, but I put in the caveat that if the test findings are negative, I do still often recommend we do a trial off of it to see if it makes a difference.

HEALING A LEAKY GUT USING THE 5 R APPROACH

1 Remove ⟶ **2** Replace ⟶ **3** Reinoculate ⟶ **4** Repair ⟶ **5** Reintroduce

This simple mnemonic, the "5 R Approach," will help you remember the process we go through to heal a leaky gut. It is the foundation of my HKHM program.

- **R**emove foods that drive inflammation
- **R**eplace vitamins, minerals, fats, fiber, protein
- **R**einoculate with prebiotics and fermented foods or a probiotic supplement plus digestive enzymes
- **R**epair with this regimen for three to six months consistently and monitor symptoms as the gut repairs itself
- **R**eintroduce foods that have been eliminated slowly, one at a time (except for the processed foods)

I will walk you through the 5 Rs, including the exact supplements I use in my practice, in section II. Barry's case is a great example of how the 5 Rs can be a powerful treatment tool.

CASE STUDY

BARRY

SYMPTOMS: CHRONIC CONSTIPATION AND ENCOPRESIS (BOWEL ACCIDENTS)

Barry was eight years old when I first met him and his mother. I was doing primary care pediatrics at the time. He had chronic constipation that had started when he was about six months of age. It was so bad that it developed into something called *encopresis*. Encopresis is when stool leaks out of the anus, soiling underwear and causing a foul odor to surround the child. Constant soiling of your underwear is embarrassing for an eight-year-old child. It also concerned me, his pediatrician, and his parents.

Encopresis can be a complex interplay among inflammation, poor nutrition, food allergies or sensitivities, emotions, or a problem with his nervous system that doesn't allow for stool to be properly eliminated.

Before coming to see me, the family had been working on this issue for years. He had seen two gastroenterologists. Those doctors prescribed Benefiber and MiraLAX, but the medications weren't working. The doctors instructed Barry's mom to increase the dosage, but it didn't solve the issue.

Barry had some bloodwork done, including environmental and food IgE allergy testing, and the results were all negative. He had not had an endoscopy or a colonoscopy. His mother's intuition told her there was something deeper to Barry's issue. She felt that the Benefiber and MiraLAX weren't addressing the underlying cause but were simply treating his symptoms.

Barry's mother eventually took him to see a naturopathic doctor (ND). From my introduction, you might recall that NDs often see patients after the conventional medical route leaves them on prescription medications but still experiencing symptoms. NDs are trained to take diet and other environmental and lifestyle factors into consideration as they create treatment plans. This ND did a full IgG food sensitivity panel on Barry. Many food results came up positive, and she advised Barry's mother to take him off those foods. She also recommended several supplements. (Food sensitivities are different from food allergies. I will cover this in more depth in chapter 4.)

Barry's mother got nervous about taking him off all those foods and brought him to see me. She wanted input from an integrative pediatrician. What I usually do in these cases is give the parents a concrete timeframe to see improvements. If Barry wasn't getting better in three months, I told her I'd recommend they return to the GI doctor to get an endoscopy and possibly a colonoscopy along with a rectal biopsy, to see if he had something called *Hirschsprung's disease* (a disease where the nerves in a child's rectum haven't formed properly). Fortunately for Barry, he did not have to get these tests.

Barry and his mother agreed to a three-month plan. We eliminated the foods his tests had shown sensitivities to on the IgG test: eggs, milk, beef, wheat, crab, pork, walnuts, peanuts, and salmon. Within two to three weeks of being off the foods, Barry's lifelong constipation nearly resolved. They were over-the-moon excited, and so was I!

One of the challenges along Barry's road to recovery was that his body no longer felt the urge to defecate. We had to get creative to help him through this. I had Mom buy him a wristwatch to remind him to go to the bathroom every two hours. Simultaneously, we gradually decreased his systemic inflammation and allowed his rectum to start working properly again. Eventually, he began to sense an impending bowel movement, and we were able to stop using his watch to remind him to go. The critical factor here was that *he* was in charge of deciding when he was ready to give up the watch. Our goal was to give him as much control over the situation as possible.

Finally, we also used supplements, a probiotic (I didn't know about the power of digestive enzymes back then), magnesium, omega-3 fats, vitamin D, and a whole food supplement. Barry's improvements happened quite rapidly; within two weeks he was no longer soiling his underwear. I often find this to be the case with kids. Once we remove whatever is triggering their inflammation, their bodies move back into balance fairly quickly, anywhere from two weeks to six months.

After the initial three months, we were able to add most of the eliminated foods back into his diet one at a time for a week at a time. He tolerated everything except the gluten and dairy. When these were added back in, the constipation returned. So we kept them out for the next six months to allow full gut healing. When we added them back after his gut was able to fully heal, he could tolerate them. However, if he ate too much pizza (gluten and dairy) all at once, or if he was eating too much dairy and gluten on a weekly basis, the constipation would return. What he was experiencing is cumulative inflammation. Too much gluten and dairy filled up his glass of inflammation too high and then he would get symptoms. However, if he was mindful and only had two pieces of pizza and didn't have any dairy or gluten for a least a week before and after their yummy pizza night, he was okay. Or if there was a birthday party or special occasion coming up and he knew he wanted to enjoy cake or Thanksgiving stuffing, he would just think ahead and set things up so he could eat it without having issues.

GARY'S CUP OF INFLAMMATION

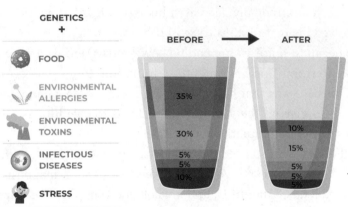

It's when we eat our inflammatory trigger foods continuously (like me in college) that we run into problems. If we don't give our system a chance to catch up and decrease the gut and systemic inflammation, it leads cumulative inflammation. (I will ask you to be mindful of cumulative inflammation when you get to the food reintroduction phase of the program.) The goal is to get the gut and system functioning well, so the kids don't have to stay on a super restrictive diet for too long. It doesn't mean eating junk food all the time. But it means understanding that the food a child eats at a typical birthday party could take their system days to recover from. Let's get their system ready for this, and if they want to partake in the pizza and cake, I would like them to be able to do it without coming home and not being able to poop for three days or vomiting with a stomachache—all of which I have seen happen with my patients after parties or after Disney World food binges!

Barry occasionally had issues with constipation (if he ate too much gluten and dairy all at once, say, in a pizza), or if he was eating it once or twice a week over several weeks. Since Barry's parents understood the concept of cumulative inflammation, they were well equipped and could always figure out the trigger behind his intermittent constipation. Together, we learned so much about what his trigger foods were that his family could plan meals and special occasion treats accordingly so Barry didn't feel deprived.

As of this writing, Barry is fifteen years old; he is five feet, eleven inches tall and thriving. He still has to watch what he eats and not ingest too much dairy and gluten. He cannot eat pizza two days in a row without having a problem (but who can, right?), and he and his family understand how to keep his bowels healthy and moving daily.

How powerful is it that Barry now understands his body so well?

A WORD ABOUT BARRY'S FOOD SENSITIVITY TESTING

Had I known when I first saw Barry what I know now, I would not have asked him to take all the foods his test results were positive for on the food sensitivity test out of his diet. I would have begun with having him remove the foods we remove during the Mini Cleanse for Kids (found in section II) along with dairy and gluten. I am pretty sure that by removing those and adding in probiotics, digestive enzymes, omega-3 fats, a whole food supplement, vitamin D, and magnesium, we would have seen the same results. I say this because I don't want anyone to think they have to run out and get a food sensitivity test done. Sometimes those tests can be more overwhelming to families than they are helpful, and their results not necessarily reproducible. (I review testing in more detail in chapter 4.)

 Research is rapidly changing

TAKEAWAYS

- The key to health is establishing a strong gut.
- The gut is the hub for about 70 percent of the immune system.
- Undigested food particles (especially protein) contribute to inflammation in the gut. When the gut is inflamed, our bodies struggle to effectively absorb nutrients from our food.
- Foods that many of us think are a healthy part of the diet may actually contribute to inflammation for some people, specifically gluten and dairy.
- Other triggers of inflammation are processed foods, artificial dyes, and refined sugar.
- Restoring integrity to the cells that line the gut (the tight junctions) is the first step in bringing your child back into balance.
- As gut inflammation decreases over time, the inflammatory symptoms start to lessen.
- Heal the gut using the 5 Rs:

(1) Remove ⟶ (2) Replace ⟶ (3) Reinoculate ⟶ (4) Repair ⟶ (5) Reintroduce

five ways food triggers inflammation in our bodies

R EWIND THE CLOCK TO the fall of 2005. I started my first job as a general pediatrician at the same practice where I had worked for three years during residency. They hired me but literally had no room in the clinic for me. So they kicked out the urologist who was renting space in the office. I took over his cubby in the back corner facing three lovely cement walls with the fourth side open to the hallway where my patient rooms were. It was perfect for a newbie. Nobody could see me sweat when I got nervous about what I was doing. And seriously . . . windows are so overrated.

One of the things I didn't learn about in training that is an ever-present part of life in a busy doctor's office is maneuvering through the many people who want to tell you about their products, including pharmaceutical reps. I was very focused on the rooms of patients who were waiting. You have three patients in rooms ready to be seen. You have a child in the middle of an asthma exacerbation getting a breathing treatment whom you saw an hour ago and you need to go back and listen to his lungs. You have a drug rep staring you down, and you have to go to the bathroom. I was still trying to find my rhythm of seeing patients, and I was not always super friendly when the reps came in during the middle of a busy clinic. Every day felt like I was stepping into a pressure cooker, but you just have to keep moving so the top doesn't blow. Many days, I barely made it to the bathroom.

However, I must recontextualize this scenario in the bigger picture of life and medicine. Healthcare workers in emergency departments, trauma centers, and hospitals and many physicians in other countries have far more stress and intensity. My job was a cakewalk compared to their intense moments of life and death. I am just giving you readers a taste of my mindset as a new doctor.

Fresh out of residency, I quickly realized that most of my patients whose illnesses were poorly controlled were struggling with the issues I am writing about in this book: reflux, eczema, recurrent ear and sinus infections, chronic runny nose, allergies, asthma, stomach pain, and constipation or loose stools (yes, I know you know this list). I was constantly writing prescriptions for increasingly stronger steroids (topical, inhaled, or ingested), antibiotics, and antacids.

Nothing about it felt right to me, and this is around the time that the voice in my head started talking to me. *"There is something else going on here! There is something you are missing, Sheila!"* I think I was subconsciously channeling my mother. I knew there was a deeper piece to this but didn't know what that piece was. I really did not like putting young children on all these medications.

Then one afternoon in the windowless corner of my office, I had a chance encounter that changed everything . . . a dark-haired Italian man walked into the clinic and our eyes locked . . . just kidding.

What really happened is a representative stopped in to talk to me. When he initially approached me in between patients, I actually thought he worked for the hospital that owned our clinic, so I didn't have my *pharmaceutical rep guard* up. This turned out to be a godsend for me and my patients because Mike worked for a company that offered allergy testing. I was intrigued immediately. You know when you hear something and you go, that is extremely important information. That's how I felt when he started talking.

He told me about a blood test on the market that would allow me to check my patients for food and environmental allergies right in the office. It was a simple blood test I could use in certain situations instead of having to refer patients to an allergist for skin-prick testing all the time. I devoured the information he gave me. I then made a follow-up call to the medical director of the company to clarify what I didn't understand and got started.

CASE STUDY

JAVIER

SYMPTOMS: STOMACHACHES AND CONSTIPATION

The first patient I used the blood allergy test on was Javier, a nine-year-old boy. He was a patient of one of the other doctors in the office, but since my partner's schedule was full, he was put on my schedule for a same-day sick visit. We new docs on the block typically have more room in our schedules to accommodate last-minute sick visits.

When Javier and his mother first came to see me, he was having terrible stomach pains and was missing a lot of school. His chart was about two inches thick (yes, we still used paper charts in those days), and while my schedule didn't permit me to read the whole thing before his visit, I spent two hours over the next two evenings going through his records.

It was eye-opening. Javier had been on seven rounds of antibiotics in just two-and-a-half years. Four of those were for strep throat, one for pneumonia, and two for sinusitis. He had also been to the clinic twice for viral gastroenteritis (diarrhea). He was now having stomachaches and was constipated on top of all of these recurrent illnesses.

I didn't understand why one child would be getting sick so often. The only thing I knew to do at that time was to start him on MiraLAX, a prescription laxative. I knew this was just a Band-Aid for the situation. My question became: how do I figure out what is *causing* not only the constipation but also his recurrent illnesses?

So I dipped my toes into the world of allergies and nutrition with Javier. General pediatrics is filled with kids who have chronic runny noses, poorly controlled eczema, and asthma, and many of them need allergy testing. I was referring one or two patients a week to the allergist. The kids would go and get their testing done and the allergist would put them on three or four meds to control their symptoms—an antihistamine, a nasal steroid spray, topical steroids for the eczema, and a stronger inhaled steroid for the asthma. Families would come back to me and not be happy with having to take so many meds.

I ordered the food and environmental allergy panels for Javier. The technical term for this bloodwork is a serum IgE panel. It looks at the same protein as skin prick tests, the test you get when you go see an allergist and they prick your back with a variety of allergens. The thought of saving patients a trip to the allergist, and a copay, and at the same time getting better continuity with the child regarding allergy treatment was very appealing.

Of course, I will always need to refer to allergists; I do not even begin to pretend I understand allergies to the depth and breadth of a trained allergist. I see myself as the first line of defense for my patients and their families.

Many things came up positive for allergies on Javier's results. Most of the foods we tested were positive, as were the environmental allergens. These results both surprised and didn't surprise me. The surprising part was that he did not have what we think of as classic environmental allergy type symptoms: runny nose, watery itchy eyes, and a cough. Instead, he had constipation, abdominal pain, and recurrent strep throat.

What started to make sense is that what he was eating and being exposed to in his environment was triggering the inflammation that was contributing to a lot of his symptoms. It gave me hope that I could help him. This is when the idea of an overflowing cup of inflammation (which you've already heard me talk about a couple of times) came to me.

JAVIER'S CUP OF INFLAMMATION

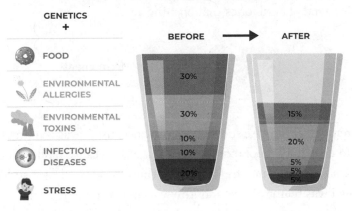

The foods that tested positive were egg white, milk, codfish, soybean, corn, and peanuts.

The environmental allergy testing results were all categorized as indoor allergens: cat, dog, cockroaches, dust mites (two different species), and mold (four different species). Molds can be found indoors and outdoors.

I gave Javier an EpiPen for the peanut allergy and referred him to a pediatric allergist to help us navigate all of these allergies. In the meantime, I asked his mother to take him off all the foods he tested positive for. I had no idea at the time how difficult it would be for the family to radically change Javier's diet. But Javier's symptoms were so severe and chronic that his mother was willing to do it.

Within a week, Javier's symptoms began to improve. I couldn't believe what I was seeing, but I also knew it was not a coincidence. His symptoms were directly related to the food he was eating. His abdominal pain resolved very quickly, and his bowel movements became easier and easier. Eventually he was having an easy daily bowel movement and we were able to wean him off the MiraLAX.

A month later Javier came in for a follow-up visit. I couldn't believe the change in him. His mother and I talked about the fact that some foods that are marketed as healthy were actually making him sick and that removing them from his diet could restore his health. The disco ball dropped once more. He continued to do great and didn't need a single round of antibiotics that ensuing year.

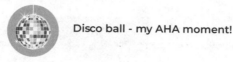

Disco ball - my AHA moment!

I remember his case so well, not only because it was the first time I had to fill out a school dietary form but also because he began to improve so quickly once he was off of those foods. All of a sudden, a family I was seeing almost monthly was not coming in as much. I was able to stay in touch with his case because of that school dietary form. (His mother had to be vigilant with the school so they would honor the changes in his diet that we were implementing, so I had to get very precise on the form, giving the cafeteria examples of what foods might contain dairy, for example.) When she saw the profound improvements in Javier's health, she was highly motivated to maintain the right nutrition for him at home and at school.

Javier's case helped me correctly deduce two things. First, once his systemic inflammation was in the right balance, his immune system could function more efficiently. Second, by decreasing the processed food he had been eating, the oppressive hold sugar had on his immune system would be lifted and he was able to move out of the sick cycle.[1]

MANY SHADES OF GRAY— FOOD ALLERGY TESTING

The more aware I became about excess inflammation in the body and how it contributed to symptoms, the more I realized how often environmental allergies and foods were part of the underlying triggers in my patients. Excess inflammation seemed to be present in about 60 to 70 percent of the kids I was seeing on a daily basis.

Understanding the interconnections among inflammation, environmental allergies, food allergies, food sensitivities, processed foods, sugar, and autoimmune diseases can make an extraordinarily large difference in the life of a patient who is suffering from anything that has to do with inflammation. And as you know by now, that's the case for most chronic illnesses.

As I continued down this path of testing kids for food allergies and advising their parents on nutrition, it quickly became apparent how gray the world of food allergy testing is compared to swabbing a child's throat and looking for the Strep bacteria. Bodily inflammation caused by foods can be triggered through several different pathways, not just the ones tested in the IgE blood or skin prick tests. For example, I might test five kids with constipation symptoms similar to Javier, but in three of them, the IgE dairy test results would be negative, despite having all the outward signs of a dairy allergy.

When the three children who didn't have positive results for an IgE dairy allergy come back for a visit, I'll explain to the parents that even though the food allergy test was negative, I still suspect dairy is playing a role in their child's issue (whether it is constipation, eczema, asthma, or chronic runny nose). We will agree on removing dairy for a short-term, doable, three-week trial while we closely monitored the child's symptoms. (You will learn how to do a gradual, selective elimination diet and how to track your child's symptoms in section II).

Seeing these kids back for their follow-ups when they are three or four weeks into their dairy-free trial is like my little mini discotheques. Not only do the common inflammatory illnesses improve, but the kids' nervous systems begin calming. Their parents tell me, "Ayisha is sleeping more soundly," or "Ahmed is more cooperative, can handle transitions better, and is having fewer meltdowns when I ask him to clean up his room." It took me several more years of studying nutrition and its many impacts to understand what was happening. It is one of the reasons it is extremely important to have concrete symptoms to track over time.

Understanding the relationship between food and inflammation and repairing that relationship in a step-by-step manner are powerful tools for helping the body heal itself. Some of the specifics of this information can be hard to process, so I created the ginormous table near the end of this chapter to help explain the many ways food can cause inflammation in our bodies. Sadly, testing for these multifaceted signs of inflammation can be confusing.

Before consulting the table, let's get on the same page with vocabulary.

FOOD ALLERGY

A food allergy is an adverse health effect arising from a specific immune response that occurs reproducibly on exposure to a given food. Once the body is sensitized to the allergen, like peanuts, minimal exposure can trigger a powerful, profound, and fast inflammatory response. Histamine is released from mast cells and this can lead to hives, lip swelling, coughing, wheezing, vomiting, and trouble breathing. The reaction typically occurs within fifteen to thirty minutes of exposure, or it can be delayed up to twelve hours. It is serious and can be life-threatening.

The following eleven foods account for about 90 percent of our food allergies and our food sensitivities. It doesn't mean these foods are unhealthy. It just means that if your child has an issue that is food related, chances are, it will involve one of these.

FOODS THAT CAUSE 90% OF FOOD ALLERGIES/ SENSITIVITIES	DAIRY	WHEAT	EGGS
CORN	SOY	PEANUTS	TREE NUTS
FISH	SHELLFISH	CITRIC ACID	SESAME

FOOD SENSITIVITY

Any symptom perceived to be related to food is referred to as a food sensitivity. Since it is subjective, food sensitivity reactions (or non-reactions) can have a wide range of interpretations. This is why I created the healthy kids happy moms - SYMPTOM TRACKER, which you'll find in section II. It is critical that we have concrete physical signs to monitor and track over time while we are changing your child's diet and adding supplements.

The best way of testing for a food sensitivity is to do a selective elimination diet, exactly what we will be doing with the HKHM program. We use our knowledge of the common foods that cause allergies and sensitivities and make some educated decisions about which foods to eliminate and in what order.

FOOD INTOLERANCE
(LACTOSE INTOLERANCE)

A food intolerance is a non-immune-mediated adverse reaction to a food and includes conditions such as lactase deficiency (lactose intolerance). Lactose intolerance, dairy allergy, and dairy sensitivity often get confused because they have so many overlapping symptoms. I see this confusion so often that it deserves some further explanation.

Lactose intolerance is when the body does not break down lactose, the sugar in dairy. It causes bloating, gas, nausea, and belly pain (see table on page 59 for symptoms). Dairy allergy is an immune-mediated reaction (which means the inflammation is triggered by cells that are part of the immune system) to one of the proteins in dairy, often casein. Casein and whey are the two main proteins in dairy. A dairy sensitivity is a non-immune-mediated reaction of the body to dairy. I will often see kids who have negative test results for a dairy allergy so parents will switch them to a lactose-free milk or formula, but their constipation, eczema, or recurrent ear or sinus infections persist. A true lactose enzyme deficiency at birth is genetic and extremely rare. Instead of being switched to a lactose-free product, these babies and young kids can do a three-week trial off casein and whey to see whether their symptoms are due to a sensitivity (which creates inflammation), to one of the proteins in dairy. Lactose-free formula and milk contains casein, so you want to use a formula that does not contain this protein. Kids one year and older can drink water or a non-dairy milk such as coconut, almond, or hemp milk.

Although most of us can break down lactose in milk at birth, we begin to lose that ability around the age of three years. As we age, our ability to break down lactose continues to decline. Globally, about 70 percent of adults are not able to break down lactose (think about the bloating and gas that ensues if you drink a milkshake).[2] The prevalence is even higher in people of South American, African, and Asian descent.

CELIAC DISEASE

This is an autoimmune disease in which the body reacts to gluten (the protein found in wheat, barley, and rye). It has a genetic component to it: once you have it, it is a lifelong condition, and you need to remain 100 percent off gluten as a new lifestyle.

HISTAMINE INTOLERANCE

Histamine is a chemical messenger in the body released when we are exposed to our allergens, both food and environmental. However, certain foods can also increase histamine release in the body, even when there is not a true allergy. The symptoms look very similar to a food allergy, but the inflammation is mediated in a different way. Some foods are simply rich in histamine, such as avocado. (I know, right? Can avocado really have any negative connotations?!)

However, other foods can actually trigger histamine to be released. I have listed all of these out in the following table so you can keep them straight. Be particularly mindful of these foods if your child has eczema flares or if you often notice flushing on them (rosy cheeks, neck, or ears) at times when they are not playing hard. Excess histamine can play a role in both of those.

For example, if your child has eczema and is already off the two big food triggers for eczema, dairy and eggs, review the list of high-histamine foods and see whether she is eating a lot of any one of them.

You may just need to cut back on that food for a few weeks, see how her skin does and, then when you add it back in, monitor once again how the skin responds.

As you read through this table, you will officially know significantly more about the many facets of food reactions than I did coming out of residency.

CATEGORY	FOOD ALLERGIES[3]	FOOD SENSITIVITIES	CELIAC DISEASE[4]
Symptoms	Flushing, hives, itching, lip swelling, coughing, trouble breathing, wheezing, abdominal pain, nausea, vomiting, diarrhea, increased heart rate	Runny nose, nasal congestion, abdominal pain, bloating, gas, loose stools or constipation, foggy brain, fatigue, skin rashes (eczema, bumps on the cheeks or back of arms), red ring around the anus, emotional outbursts, trouble focusing	Weight loss or weight gain, poor growth in children (short stature, failure to thrive), abdominal pain, bloating, gas, chronic loose stools or constipation, foggy brain, fatigue, trouble sleeping, joint or bone pain, iron-deficient anemia, B12 deficiency, menstrual irregularities, infertility, skin rash (dermatitis herpetiformis), behavior challenges, meltdowns or mood swings, trouble focusing, ADHD, anxiety, depression, seizures, numbness or tingling in the hands and feet
Speed of Reaction	Usually within fifteen minutes to two hours (but can be delayed up to twelve hours)	Minutes to hours to days	Symptoms can be extremely gradual and insidious. It often takes individuals years to get the right diagnosis (97 percent of people who have celiac disease do not know it, and the prevalence is 1 in 133)[5]

CATEGORY	FOOD ALLERGIES[3]	FOOD SENSITIVITIES	CELIAC DISEASE[4]
Cells Involved	Immune system IgE	Non-immune system	Immune system IgA and T-cells
Food Examples	Peanut Tree nuts Milk Egg Soy Wheat Corn Fish Shellfish Citric acid Sesame	Milk Egg Soy Wheat (gluten) Corn Citric acid Sesame	Gluten (the protein found in barley, wheat, and rye and many other processed foods)
Testing	Skin prick test *or* Bloodwork	Selective elimination diet Blood test is controversial: many food sensitivity tests are available that test for IgG proteins to various foods. Some research suggests that elevated IgG4 proteins confer "tolerance" to a food	Blood test for antibodies TTG (IgA, IgG) DGP (IgA, IgG) EMA(IgA) Endoscopy with biopsy of the small intestine to look for damage **Must be eating gluten for the testing to be accurate**
Gold Standard Test	Oral Food Challenge	Selective elimination diet followed by reintroduction of the food (the HKHM program)	Endoscopy with biopsy

An Oral Food Challenge (OFC) is a medical procedure in which a food is eaten slowly, in gradually increasing amounts, under medical supervision, to accurately diagnose or rule out a true food allergy.

TYPE OF REACTIONS	FOOD INTOLERANCE[6]	HISTAMINE INTOLERANCE
Symptoms/Disease	**Lactase deficiency (lactose intolerance):** bloating, gas, abdominal pain, nausea with ingestion of dairy **Allergic colitis:** babies will present with blood in their stool **Eosinophilic esophagitis (EE):** discomfort in the upper chest and esophagus while eating; sometimes leads to avoiding eating **Food protein-induced entero-colitis syndrome (FPIES):** vomiting and diarrhea after ingesting certain foods in babies	Similar to allergy symptoms: Flushing of the face, neck, ears, and body (can make eczema worse) Nausea Burning in the mouth Headache Faintness Abdominal cramps Bloating Diarrhea Wheezing or other breathing problems Swelling of the face and tongue
Speed of Reaction	Can be rapid or within hours	Often within minutes to hours but can also persist if histamine levels remain elevated.
Cells Involved	Non-immune system Non-IgE mediated Cellular reaction Even though these issues seem similar to food allergies, most often the standard IgE food test results will be negative for cow's milk even though it can be contributing to the inflammation	Non-immune system When the diamine oxidase (DAO) enzyme which breaks down histamine in our bodies is not functioning properly
Food Examples	**EE: common triggers** Milk Eggs Soy Wheat Others **FPIES: common triggers** Milk	**Histamine-rich foods** Spoiled fish Cured or smoked meats Smoked or canned fish Shellfish Leftover meats Fermented food (including beer) Vinegar Cow's milk, yogurt Cheeses, aged cheeses

Food Examples (continued)	Soy Rice Chicken Others	Avocado Eggplant Spinach **Foods that trigger histamine release** Bananas Citrus fruits (lemons, oranges) Cherries Pineapple Strawberries Dried fruit Tomatoes Tree nuts Legumes (peanuts, beans) Chocolate Wheat germ Food dyes, additives, and some seasonings Alcohol
Testing	Doctor will decide based upon history, symptoms, and physical exam Possibly test stool for blood or perform endoscopy for abnormal cells (EE)	Doctor will decide based upon history, symptoms, circumstances when the symptoms occur, and physical exam

If I were to see Javier for the first time now, I would have much better and more concrete instructions to help his family get started. The steps outlined in section II of this book are the ones I developed over the past fifteen plus years of seeing hundreds of patients just like Javier.

Today when I am evaluating a patient similar to Javier in my clinic, I do the IgE environmental allergy test when appropriate based upon symptoms. If I suspect a true food allergy, I generally refer to a pediatric allergist. If I don't suspect a true food allergy, I test the child for celiac disease and then proceed with gradually removing dairy over three to four weeks and then removing gluten the same way.

> You must be eating gluten when testing for celiac disease. Once you remove it from your child's diet for several months, or possibly even weeks, even if they have celiac disease, the antibodies may convert to being negative and you would get a false negative result. The child may actually have celiac disease, but the antibodies are not showing up because the food is no longer triggering a reaction in the body.

Research in the field of nutrition is rapidly growing. I continue to expand my toolbox about how best to advise parents. One area that remains consistent is that certain foods drive inflammation. Inflammation hinders the immune system and also impacts many other systems of the body in addition to the gut, skin, lungs, sinuses, and ears. Typically, the kids who have the most profound improvements with nutrition changes are the ones who present with a constellation of inflammatory symptoms.

As I used this concept that inflammation drives illness to look for the root cause of symptoms, it revolutionized my practice. I revised all my carefully crafted handouts not only to include the medications we might need for acute symptoms but also to educate families about how to decrease their exposure to specific allergens, how to look at nutrition to optimize natural anti-inflammatory foods, and how to remove foods that can be extremely pro-inflammatory. It continues to be eye-opening for me how environmental allergy symptoms improve when one cleans up the diet.

TAKEAWAYS

- True food allergy is mediated by the immune system (like a peanut allergy). It's diagnosed through a blood or skin prick test, patient history, and physical examination.
- Food sensitivity is an inflammation created by food, but not a true allergy. It's diagnosed through a selective elimination diet.

- Celiac disease is an autoimmune allergy to gluten, the protein found in wheat, barley, and rye. It's diagnosed through bloodwork or an endoscopy with biopsy. You can have celiac disease but not have an IgE wheat allergy.
- Food intolerance is inflammation along the GI tract which is mediated by food, but not a true allergy. Lactose intolerance is an example. It's diagnosed in conjunction with your healthcare provider.
- Histamine intolerance is a reaction to foods that increase histamine levels, where the body is not efficiently able to break down and clear the histamine. It's not a true allergy. It's diagnosed in conjunction with your healthcare provider.
- Testing and diagnosing food reactions is not always straightforward. But as you begin to understand some of the subtle differences in how foods can affect us, you will understand why the HKHM program in section II is laid out the way that it is.

CHAPTER 5

overfed and undernourished

T HE FIRST TIME I became aware that artificial dyes and preservatives could impact children's behavior and health was in 2010. Eleven-year-old Adam, who had ADHD, came to see me. His mother told me that when Adam ate food or candy with blue dye, he'd flap his hands like a child on the autism spectrum, and when he ingested caramel coloring, he would sniff his fingers.

I had never heard of anything like this. I listened intently and then looked to see whether there was any research on this phenomenon.

What was happening to Adam? Caramel coloring is made from food sources, such as wheat, barley, or milk, and milk is the most common source.[1] Each of these individual foods are common allergens, so Adam could have had a sensitivity to one of these foods and not the caramel coloring itself.

This mother was quite certain there was a direct correlation. Although it took her a while to figure it out, she had tested her hypothesis. She had given Adam those colorings on several occasions and watched his physical movements change. Adam was a gregarious young fella, and he understood how these ingredients impacted him. He explained that he would know he had accidentally ingested these ingredients because he would start flapping his hands or smelling his fingertips. He didn't like feeling of being out of control of his body and was more than willing to avoid them.

Mom had him on an all-organic diet free of artificial dyes, preservatives, gluten, and dairy prior to seeing me, and he was doing great. She brought him in for a well visit and as we talked through his history, she shared these things with me. I was blown away. Like Adam's mother, many families can make nutrition changes at home and not need any further in-depth testing by a pediatrician.

WHEN AND HOW DID FOOD BECOME PROBLEMATIC?

Over the years, I've seen many kids whose parents have witnessed drastic changes in behavior after consuming certain dyes and additives. Since it can be challenging to decipher specifically what foods are triggering certain behaviors, I recommend you keep all or at least most artificial dyes and food preservatives out of your child's diet.

What makes this difficult is that we have received nutritional advice and heavy marketing that has been driven less by what is the healthiest for our bodies and more by what is available and can be easily mass produced. We are extremely fortunate in this country to have an abundant food supply, but we still have millions of kids who go to bed hungry every night. We have another set of kids who are overfed and undernourished because of what they are eating. Too much of what we call food today isn't real food, despite the marketing. It is greatly altered from what is found in nature.

A popular chip was invented in 1964 and on the national market in 1966; the chips include artificial colors (including Yellow 6, Yellow 5, and Red 40) and chemicals the average person cannot pronounce. The ingredients have changed over the years and vary based upon flavor, so read the labels!

A sports drink was created in 1965 to help the University of Florida football players keep up their hydration, electrolytes, and carbohydrate levels during football games in the extreme Florida heat. It proved to make a significant difference in the athletic performance of these elite athletes. It seems now, however, that our young children play thirty minutes of soccer, maybe break a slight sweat, and then we give them bottles of a rehydration solution developed for elite athletes performing in 80- to 100-degree temperatures. Many sports drinks hit the categories we are aiming to remove: excess refined sugar, artificial dyes, and preservatives. Check out the ingredients of a popular lemon-lime sports drink: Water, Sugar, Dextrose, Citric Acid, Salt, Sodium Citrate, Monopotassium Phosphate, Gum Arabic, Glycerol Ester of Rosin, Natural Flavor, Yellow 5.

How did we come to this point of eating and drinking such non-foods? World War II created a need for packaged food to support soldiers on the battlefield. In this same timeframe, many American women entered the workforce, pulling them away from the kitchen. Many women continued to work after the war ended, and packaged food became a common commodity in the American diet. Working mothers have often taken the blame for our era of packaged food, and that is so far from reality.

After World War II, when munition factories transitioned from war production to consumer production, the world was suddenly in need of something to do with all that unused nitrogen. It didn't take long to convince farmers to grow crops faster and more abundantly by applying nitrogen-based fertilizers instead of the manure and "cover crops" they traditionally used to enrich the soil. Almost overnight, we had a surplus of corn, which we turned into corn oil and corn-based packaged foods. High fructose corn syrup is in so many products— everything from salad dressing and ketchup to cereal, breads, and crackers to sodas and sports drinks.

Grain crops, such as wheat and oats, also became more plentiful after World War II, often running to surplus. It isn't difficult to draw a line between grain surplus and the federal government's emphasis on grains in the American diet. When the United States Department of Agriculture (USDA) started recommending dietary standards in 1946, grains got the lion's share of daily recommended servings and dairy enjoyed its status as an entire food group. Nuts were nowhere to be found.

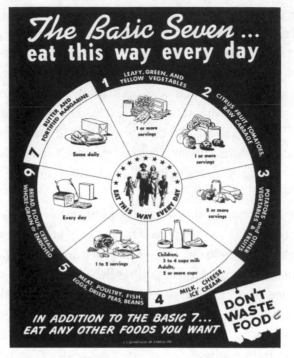

Photo courtesy of National Archives and Records Administration, September 1946.

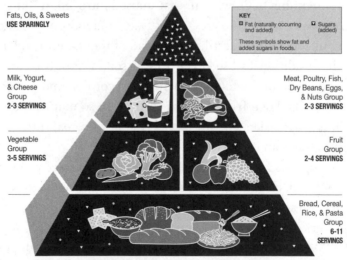

The food guide pyramid. Food and Nutrition Service, US Department of Agriculture.

From 1992 to 2005, the USDA represented ideal consumption with a food pyramid that once again emphasized grains. Dairy kept its own food group. On the bright side, nuts got mentioned in the protein group.

MyPlate replaced the USDA's MyPyramid guide on June 2, 2011. It gives equal weight to vegetables and grains. Note dairy remains the recommended drink.

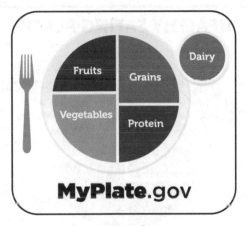

USDA MyPlate.

As you'll see in later chapters, the HKHM program emphasizes leafy greens, cruciferous vegetables, fruits, fiber (through seeds, nuts, and legumes), healthy fats, unprocessed fats, unprocessed proteins, and plain water.

While the guidelines have always included agribusiness and the food processor lobby, these interests have been gaining the upper hand over the scientists. This space between science and big business is one I have been trying to understand for many years. But wading through the research details of government food recommendations and who is making them and who is sitting on those committees can be daunting. Imagine my delight when the hallowed halls of Harvard tackled the matter. Using scientific trials, their School of Public Health confirmed what I have seen in my own practice and sheds light onto a topic fraught with gray once I began better to understand food and inflammation.

Check out this chart, starting with the glass of water in the place where we're accustomed to seeing cow's milk. Notice that vegetables dominate the plate, followed by healthy protein. They followed 100,000 nurses and health professionals for up to twelve years and used a questionnaire to track their diets. The results are impressive.[2,3]

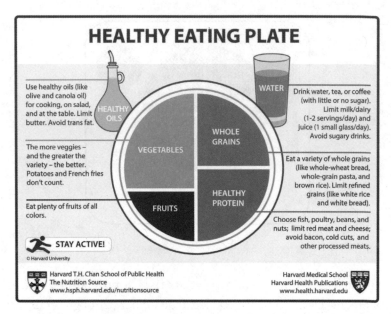

Copyright © 2011 Harvard University. For more information about The Healthy Eating Plate, please see The Nutrition Source, Department of Nutrition, Harvard T.H. Chan School of Public Health, http://www.thenutritionsource.org and Harvard Health Publications, health.harvard.edu.

- Those who most closely followed the US Government's Food Pyramid guidelines reduced their overall risk of developing heart disease, cancer, or other chronic disease by 11 percent for men and 3 percent for women.
- Those whose diets most closely followed Harvard's Healthy Eating Plate lowered their risk of heart disease in men by almost 40 percent and women by almost 30 percent.

My HKHM program tracks with the Harvard recommendations. If your gut has been telling you all the milk, pasta, pizza, and mac and cheese that your child eats might not be great for them even though that's what we serve them in schools and restaurants, your gut is onto something.

MINI CLEANSE FOR KIDS— MAKE ROOM FOR HEALTHY FOODS

I recommend a system of eating for your family that involves more vegetables, fruits, and other high-fiber foods such as nuts and seeds, in addition to healthy fats and proteins. The first step in this journey is to make room for healthy foods and drinks that will help reduce your child's inflammation, which we will discuss in chapter 6.

Details on how to succeed with the Mini Cleanse are found in section II, while section III includes recipes that will please and appease your child's taste buds. What follows here is a brief overview of the ingredients I want you to avoid—and why.

SUGAR AND CHILDREN'S HEALTH

 Almost 20 percent of US children between the ages of two and nineteen are obese.[4] Sugary drinks are the leading sources of added sugars in the American diet. On any given day, 63 percent of kids and 49 percent of adults drink a sugar-sweetened beverage.[5] The excess sugar intake is associated with the following.

- Weight gain/obesity
- Type 2 diabetes
- Heart disease
- Kidney diseases
- Non-alcoholic liver disease
- Tooth decay and cavities
- Gout (in adults)
- Arthritis[6]
- Hindered brain function[7,8]

By simply removing one sugar-filled drink daily (for many of your children this might be eliminating fruit juices), you can remove an inflammatory, immune-suppressant roadblock that may be holding your child in the sick cycle.

According to Harvard School of Public Health, "If current US trends continue, more than 57 percent of today's youth will be obese at age thirty-five."[9] I seldom talk about weight loss in kids, as I prefer to focus on healthy food as fuel for the body and brain. As children begin eating foods that are better for their systems, they continue to grow taller but stop gaining weight at the same rate they had been. This keeps the discussion away from weight loss and instead about the foods that work best for their systems.

ARTIFICIAL COLORS AND BEHAVIOR

 Many of you have experienced your child's behavior shifts with dyes. Avoid FD&C Red No. 40 or FD&C Yellow No. 5. FD&C stands for Food, Drug & Cosmetics. There are many FD&C colors, and they're found in everything.

Since 2010 in the United Kingdom, food products that contain artificial dyes are required to have a warning label stating that the food "may have an adverse effect on activity and attention in children." Because of this ruling, certain US based companies voluntarily removed artificial dyes from their products in the UK and Europe, but not in the US.

The impact of artificial dyes and colors on children's health and behavior has long been debated in the pediatric world, but cases as far back as the mid-1970s linked food additives—and dyes particularly—to behavior and learning disorders. Ben Feingold, MD, studied 1,200 children and the impact that 3,000 different food additives had on their health and behavior. He shared the results of this study in his book, *The Feingold Diet: Why Your Child Is Hyperactive.*

Feingold identified a link between children's behavior and certain foods (such as dairy and wheat), artificial dyes, colors, and preservatives, as well as compounds such as salicylic acids. Dr. Feingold's work remains controversial because of inconsistencies in the study results.

My stance is that if we can get kids to eat better food with fewer additives, let's do it!

PROCESSED FOODS ARE INFLAMMATORY

Once you become aware of the excessive sugar in packaged foods, you'll understand how kids' taste buds are bathed in sugar. These taste buds may then flat-out reject leafy green vegetables or foods filled with healthy fats, including olives, olive oil, avocado, almonds, walnuts, and fermented foods such as sauerkraut, which is rich in probiotics.

Sugar is everywhere, from organic, non-GMO (genetically modified organisms) "health foods" to highly processed, chemical-laden foods, like packaged children's candies. The food industry hides sugar under many different names ending with the suffix -ose. The more classic sugars are as follows.

Dextrose	Glucose solids
Fructose	High-fructose corn syrup
Galactose	Lactose
Fruit juice concentrate	Maltose
Glucose	Sucrose

Artificial sweeteners should also be avoided. They can negatively impact the beneficial bacteria in the gut.[10]

Saccharin (Sweet'N Low)
Sucralose (Splenda)
Aspartame (NutraSweet, Equal)
Neotame (Newtame)
Acesulfame potassium or ace-K (Sweet One)

If your child has a significant sweet tooth, consider sw
more natural sweetener, such as honey, maple syrup, bla
lasses, or monk fruit.

PROCESSED MEATS

 Hot dogs and processed meats have become a staple for many children. The nitrates in processed meats are extremely damaging to our heart and blood vessels.[11,12,13,14,15]
Hardened arteries are not something we think of in young children, but if you can bring better balance to their processed meat intake, making it a treat instead of the norm, you will make great strides in providing healthier, less inflammatory proteins for your child's system. Reducing this inflammatory ingredient will lower their cardiovascular risk.

PROCESSED FATS

 Most processed foods are made with these oils, which are inflammatory in and of themselves. When they are used at high heat, they become even more inflammatory and increase your child's cup of inflammation. You should try to avoid:

Canola oil	Safflower oil
Grapeseed oil	Soybean oil
Rice bran oil	Corn oil
"Vegetable" oil	Cottonseed oil

TRUE CONFESSION:
I Used to Eat Candy Bars for Breakfast

I'll never forget the winter of 2005. I was a third-year pediatric resident exhausted both emotionally and physically. I wanted an "easy" rotation, where I didn't have to take any overnight call. I also wanted to spend some time with my family out West. I knew my parents would feed and take care of me while I refueled for my last several months of residency, so I organized a rotation in Seattle at Bastyr University.

Bastyr is one of four schools in the US that trains naturopathic doctors. The curriculum for a doctorate in naturopathic medicine is roughly parallel to that of traditional medical schools. Students put in the same hours as conventional medical students in terms of course-load, but they also learn about nutrition, herbs, supplements, mind-body therapies, and other natural treatments.

Part of my interest in natural therapies stemmed from my yoga practice, which I'd started during medical school. Yoga opened my eyes to a whole different way of being. Once I realized how much better I could feel because of this practice, it made me wonder about other healthy lifestyle practices.

My interest in natural medicine likely originated during childhood. My parents raised my four siblings and me in as natural a way as possible in Avon Lake, Ohio, a suburb of Cleveland. We grew a huge vegetable garden during the summer, which covered almost every square inch of our backyard. My siblings and I grew up eating fresh food.

My parents later moved to Bainbridge Island, a thirty-five-minute ferry ride from downtown Seattle. Since the Bastyr clinic was in Seattle, I'd wake at the crack of dawn, catch a ferry with my brother-in-law, and then take a cab to the clinic in Ballard, a neighborhood not far from the ferry terminal in downtown Seattle.

Snickers bar and Diet Coke in my backpack, I was naively ready for what I expected would be my easy month rotation of no overnight call and learning what naturopathic doctors do.

In the morning, the students met to discuss patients in a small, nondescript conference room, cluttered with books and papers, with just enough room for seven or eight of us.

When I arrived, I noticed that everyone was drinking herbal tea and eating healthy-looking whole-grain muffins. I was too embarrassed to pull out my Diet Coke and Snickers bar. I looked longingly at the whole-grain muffins and mugs filled with lovely smelling teas. I thought, *How can I get my hands on one of those muffins?*

By lunchtime I was so hungry I had a headache, and I realized I needed to make a few changes. The first was obvious: I had to give up my beloved Diet Coke. In college, my girlfriends and I would make special trips to convenience stores with the best fountain drinks. A thirty-two-ounce Diet Coke wasn't out of the ordinary for me. We went so far as to figure out which restaurants had the best crushed ice that made the Diet Coke taste even better. The amount of Diet Coke we drank in those days was impressive. And now, that love affair was about to come to an abrupt end.

I didn't touch another Diet Coke that month, and I had a raging headache for most of the month. I'm not one who gets headaches often, so I wasn't sure what was happening to me. I continued to consume caffeine, replacing my Diet Coke habit with black tea, yet I still was popping three or four ibuprofen several times a week.

Sadly, that was the first time I stopped and asked myself, *What the heck is* in *this black, carbonated liquid?*

When I finally got the courage to start speaking up in this clinic, I pointed out the complexity of the patients' cases compared to the more run-of-the-mill patients I was used to seeing. The number of specialty doctors these patients had seen, and the amount of testing they'd endured, floored me. Not to mention the thousands of dollars these patients had spent on medical bills or the time consumed. And for what? They didn't feel better.

Throughout the month, I continued to be impressed by how much the naturopathic doctors understood about nutrition and its impact on health, and I often had no idea what they were talking about. Food sensitivity this, food sensitivity that . . . . *Your school has a nutritionist who takes people on grocery store tours? What does nutrition have to do with any of this?*

I laugh now when I think about how easy I thought this rotation would be. In some ways, it was more challenging than any of my previous rotations. I wasn't on call and having to stay awake every fourth night, but the cases that came into that clinic were extremely complicated. These patients were doing everything their medical doctor had recommended, but they still struggled.

At Bastyr, it was as if the top of my head opened up and streams of new information poured in. I didn't realize how that month would profoundly impact my own health, my career, my outlook, and the hundreds of patients I'd eventually care for.

When I returned to Charlotte, I still had several months of residency, so I tabled all the new information. I had no idea how to incorporate it into the hospital setting, which is where most of residency takes place. The food served to hospital patients would make many healthy people ill. Jell-O, pudding, macaroni and cheese—come on, really?

I kept my head in the sand for a few more months, but then, when I was finally seeing my own patients in a regular clinic, I started to put everything together. Today, when I'm thinking through a child's health issue, my brain starts to write a recipe for reducing their inflammation.

As I've told you already, the first part of reducing inflammation is removing inflammatory ingredients. The second part is adding foods and supplements that support the body's natural healing mechanisms. We will delve into these healing foods next.

TAKEAWAY

I will give you a quote from Michael Pollen, who has written many books on food and the food industry: "Eat real food, mostly plants, and not too much."

CHAPTER 6

focus foods: fats, fiber, and protein

IN OUR SOCIETY, MANY of our children are overfed yet undernourished. Diets high in simple carbs, dairy, and meats leave little room for the healthy foods I prefer your children eat. The nutrient-rich foods we are talking about in this chapter include vegetables, seeds, nuts, and beans, along with fats, fiber, and protein options aplenty.

In chapter 5, I asked you to eliminate a myriad of tasty, sugary foods with the promise that I'd provide you with plenty of alternatives. Little by little, your child's taste buds will begin to enjoy different foods. (You'll find some of my favorite kid-friendly recipes in section III.)

What's that I hear you saying? Your child is a picky eater who will never try new foods? Cassie's case will inspire you to give the HKHM program your best effort.

• • •

CASSIE

SYMPTOMS: ECZEMA AND A PICKY EATER

Cassie was about two-and-a-half years old when her mom first brought her to see me. Cassie was this super-bright, mischievous girl with a huge smile, light brown hair, pale skin, and profound dark circles under her eyes. She also had significant eczema and constipation and was an extremely picky eater.

Her parents had already figured out she was allergic to milk before coming to see me, so she wasn't drinking cow's milk. Instead she was drinking thirty-two ounces of soy milk daily. When she originally went off the cow's milk, months before they came to see me, her eczema improved but didn't fully resolve. She'd had skin prick testing for environmental allergens and was allergic to cats, dogs, dust mites, and pigweed and was such an extremely picky eater (she only ate about seven or eight foods) and had so many food allergies (here is her list: egg whites, almonds, Brazil nuts, cashews, coconut, hazelnut, peanuts, pecans, pistachios, and walnuts) that the GI doctor did an endoscopy on her to be sure she didn't have something called eosinophilic esophagitis (EE), an allergic condition of the esophagus, an ulcer, or celiac disease. She did not have any of those, and despite the limited foods she would eat, she continued to grow and gain weight beautifully.

Fortunately, Cassie stayed on her growth curve each year at her pediatric well visits, and I think she was likely sustained by the volume and calories she was getting from the soy milk. I mention this here because if your child is underweight or losing weight, this program is not the right fit for you at this time. You don't want to decrease their calorie intake unless they are being closely monitored by your child's doctor and possibly a feeding therapist or a registered dietician.

Before making any changes with Cassie, I did some lab work

and started her on the foundational supplements. The bloodwork was to look for nutrient deficiencies. Her hemoglobin was normal, so she was not anemic, but her iron stores (as measured by a ferritin) and iron saturation were quite low. Therefore we could deduce that she was not eating an adequate amount of iron and that her body was not absorbing what she was eating efficiently.

We also looked at her zinc; magnesium; copper; vitamins D, B_{12}, and B_6; as well as her blood counts. Her zinc was surprisingly normal given the fact that zinc levels tend to be lower with 'picky eaters.' I did not start iron with her at this time because we needed to first decrease the inflammation in her gut and begin to optimize digestion with the foundational supplements (probiotic, digestive enzymes, omega-3 fats, a whole foods supplement, and vitamin D). Otherwise, she likely would not absorb the iron from the supplement well either.

Cassie began to have small improvements with the supplements, but I knew we needed to get her off the soy milk. I suspected that was also part of her systemic inflammation and might be part of what was still triggering her eczema. I also wanted her to begin eating more nutrient-rich foods instead of drinking so many calories through a plant-based beverage.

Over the next several months, Cassie's mom was able to wean her completely to water plus eight to ten ounces per day of some of other plant-based beverages. Cassie still was not eating a whole lot of fresh foods; she subsisted on packaged snack foods that were mainly carbs and the omega-6 vegetable fats. The inflammatory/sick cycle was not going to be broken until we could get her ingesting (through food and supplements) more omega-3 fats, vitamins, and minerals. As we decreased her calories from the soy milk, her appetite picked up slightly because she was starting to feel hunger cues. It's another disco ball moment when the gut-brain connection wakes up. The gut-brain wakeup happens as cellular health improves. The wakeup is when your picky eater says they're hungry and will actually eat something besides their go-to packaged snack.

cow's milk vs. soy beverage (soy milk)

A high percentage of kids who are allergic or sensitive to cow's milk may also be sensitive to soy (at least initially when their systems are so inflamed). I learned this the hard way, unfortunately. When I first started working with families to remove cow's milk from their children's diets, we would invariably switch kids from cow's milk to a soy beverage. Then six weeks later, the kids would come back to the office with diarrhea, irritability, or a different type of rash. For this reason, when I remove dairy from kids' diets, we don't replace twenty-four ounces of cow's milk with twenty-four ounces of soy beverage (or another type of non-dairy milk). Rather, we switch them to water if possible, and then, if the child loves drinking milk, they can drink eight to ten ounces per day of a non-dairy plant-based beverage (such as hemp, coconut, oat, or tree nut).

Timing is key. You can't force the timing of this wakeup. We let the supplements do the work at first (primarily the probiotics and digestive enzyme) so the child feels better, in part because their bowels are working better. The gradual decrease in soy milk allows us to decrease calories safely and without too much emotional stress that you might feel when taking away a primary food source from your child. Using this method gives everyone ample time to figure out what the kids *will* eat.

When Cassie had a slightly better appetite, we partnered the family with Haynes, the health coach in our practice. Haynes met Cassie and her mother at the farmer's market and talked through different ways to start inspiring Cassie to try some new foods. Haynes went over some of the recipes in section III (many of which Haynes contributed!).

I got a message later that day that Cassie sat down and ate almost an entire tray of baked kale. She had never touched anything like that before: it was one step on a journey to getting her to eat nutrients so she would be able to supply her cells with what they needed instead of having to rely so heavily on the supplements. She continued to eat more and more foods and mom learned new ways to encourage Cassie to eat more vegetables and high-fiber foods. If we had pushed the vegetables on Cassie too soon, her system might not have accepted them so readily.

Once Cassie was fully off the soy milk, the eczema on her body cleared. However, despite being on great supplements and improving nutrition, she continued to have an area just around her mouth that would flare up several times a month. And during the rest of the month, she just had small pinkish papules scattered around her mouth. We eventually figured out they had some previous water damage in their home and mold had grown in that area. Once we realized that, the parents brought in a certified mold expert who tested the mold first and then had a different company, also mold-certified, do the remediation. Once that was complete, the flares around her mouth resolved, as did several of mom's health issues. We were able to pull Cassie off most of her supplements other than the foundational ones and she continues to do great to this day! No further eczema, peri-oral mouth rash, or constipation, and she is a much more adventurous eater—no sushi and caviar, but she eats more veggies! (See the appendix and my website for further information if you suspect any water damage or mold in your home.)

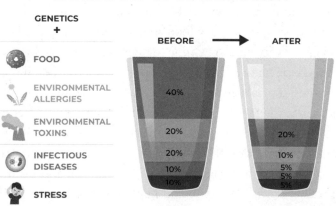

CASSIE'S CUP OF INFLAMMATION

GENETICS
+

FOOD

ENVIRONMENTAL ALLERGIES

ENVIRONMENTAL TOXINS

INFECTIOUS DISEASES

STRESS

BEFORE → AFTER

BEFORE: 40%, 20%, 20%, 10%, 10%

AFTER: 20%, 10%, 5%, 5%, 5%

HEALTHY FATS, HEALTHY KIDS

Cassie is a good example of a child who was not eating many of the right fats initially, so her cell walls were not as healthy as they could have been. If our cell walls do not contain the right balance of fats (enough omega-3 fats), it is much more difficult to get our skin and guts into balance because they depend upon the health of each of the individual cells. This brings me to discuss a much-maligned food group: fats.

When the processed food industry talks to us about fats, they bury us under a deluge of words like saturated/unsaturated and even mono-saturated and polyunsaturated. It's not as complicated as we've been led to believe. When talking about fats, we need to talk about the balance of fats in our diets. The standard American diet is heavy in omega-6 and -9 fats and low in omega-3 fats.

Foods rich in omega-3 fats are *never* marketed to children. It's a short list, and your kids probably don't eat many of these foods regularly.

OMEGA-3 FOODS
Coldwater fish: salmon, mackerel, herring, trout, char, sockeye, sardines
Flaxseeds, flax oil
Chia seeds
Hemp seeds
Walnuts
Almonds
Berries: blackberries, blueberries, strawberries
Brussels sprouts and other green leafy vegetables
Eggs (free range)
Grass-fed beef, lamb, and wild game such as venison

Some of these foods contain both omega-3 and omega-6 fats.

While fats have gotten a bad rap, they're *extremely* important for all of us, especially the developing brain of a baby, both in utero and after birth. Every cell in our body has a fat layer called a *phospholipid bilayer*, and many of the health issues I see in kids, from eczema to asthma, are related in part to a lack of healthy fats in the child's diet.[1]

Because fats make up our cell walls, they are responsible for proper cellular integrity so nutrients can move in and out of the cells fluidly.[2] Healthy cell walls also facilitate cell-to-cell signaling, directly or indirectly through neurotransmitters, hormones, and even medications. Cell signal transmission is critical for almost every system of our body, from our nervous system, doing math homework and being able to calm ourselves down, to sending hormonal messages (going through puberty, muscle growth), to our beating heart cells and our immune system.

To better understand cell-to-cell signaling, think about your internet connection: when there is a storm, your internet connection is not as good because the signal gets dampened by the weather. It is the same in the body: If we have too much inflammation, the chemical signals have to wade through excess body inflammation and we don't get great signal transmission.

Improving the makeup of the cell walls happens over time. In our practice we affectionately refer to this shift as an oil change for the kids' cell walls. It can be a slow process, but if we stick with it, we see the long-lasting results. For Cassie, she was eating fats but too many of the wrong type of fats from the abundant omega-6 vegetable oils in the packaged snack foods. I see this in most of my little patients. Today's kids eat so many of these processed foods that it leaves little room in their diet for the good stuff. But have no fear, as you go through the Mini Cleanse, it will open up an enjoyable path in your child's daily intake for more of the beneficial fats.

healthy fats and ADHD

If you have healthy cells with the correct omega-6 to omega-3 ratio and need to be on any medication—from steroids, to antibiotics, to anti-anxiety meds, or stimulants for ADHD—the medication will likely be able to do its job more easily, at the lowest dose possible, with the fewest side effects.[3,4]

I'm not going to spend a lot of time discussing attention issues in this book, but perhaps you see the connection I'm making among healthy fats, healthy brains, and a child's capacity to calm down and to focus. I recommend omega-3 fat supplements for most of the children in my practice who are on stimulant medication for attention deficit and hyperactivity disorder to optimize their ratio of omega-6 to omega-3 fats.

Has your child ever had to go on an antibiotic for an ear infection, and it didn't clear up on the first round of medicine? And you subsequently had to go back to the pediatrician and get one, maybe two or more rounds of more potent antibiotics? This may be due to antibiotic-resistant bacteria, but if your child's cells have the correct balance of fats (with enough omega-3 fats) and minimal systemic inflammation, her immune system may be better equipped to clear the infection.

Understanding cellular health and inflammation in this way, consider how you might begin to change the course of your child's health and immune system. Eating a balanced diet will allow her immune system to work like the beautiful and complex orchestra that it is. The medication then doesn't have to wade through all that inflammation to get the job done. Imagine that if your child's immune system is so effective and efficient because of adequate fats and the other nutrients we'll review in this book, she wouldn't even succumb to the ear infection in the first place. Isn't that an exciting prospect?

SPECIAL FAT CONSIDERATIONS
FOR CHILDREN WITH ASTHMA

As I write about the role that healthy fats play in reversing the inflammatory cascade, I see the sweet faces of children I have seen over the years with significant asthma and dark circles under their eyes. Their systems at baseline have a genetic predisposition to overreact to invaders (viruses, secondhand smoke, allergens, or whatever their individual asthma triggers are). When you add processed foods and lots of inflammatory fats on top of these triggers, the dangerous combination results in frequent asthma attacks that require higher and higher doses of steroids to bring them under control, and subsequently higher doses of daily inhaler medications to hold their excessive baseline inflammation at bay.

> Many kids who have stuck to the HKHM program have gone from frequent asthma attacks, frequent oral steroid courses needed—and even frequent hospitalizations—to enjoying months without ever having to use their rescue inhalers while we gradually decrease the amount of daily inhaled steroid they needed in order to keep their inflammation at bay. We wean them from their medications slowly, safely, and in conjunction with their pulmonologist or allergist. Altering your child's asthma medications is absolutely not something to do on your own.

The cup of inflammation for a child with asthma is quite full. The inhaled or oral steroids keep the inflammation at bay, but they don't actually decrease the cup of inflammation, which is why these medications are needed on a daily basis. A child who is no longer living in fear of an asthma attack around every corner, and whose body has minimal inflammation, is a different child from the one requiring a rescue inhaler several times a week. I use the integrative approach by using medications to hold inflammation at bay, while we decrease the child's systemic inflammation using food and supplements. In time, dark circles under the eyes improve, eczema improves, the steroid bloat resolves, and their coloring is better.

The intangible shifts are actually the ones that I think about as I write this. When a child has an asthma attack, it is like going from breathing through a big fat straw to breathing out of a cocktail straw in a matter of minutes. The gift of working with these children and their families through their illness is beyond any professional satisfaction I could have ever imagined.

GET FIBER FROM PLANT-BASED FOODS

Fats require strong digestion to break them down into their component parts so that they may be repurposed into the many critical functions I listed above. Fiber will help rebuild the body's digestive power and is a key component to gut health.

Fiber is classified into two types, *soluble* and *insoluble*. Both are vital. Fiber lowers cholesterol, manages blood sugar, keeps the bowels regular and, best of all, it ferments in the colon and provides prebiotics—food for the healthy bacteria in the gut. As a culture, we have gotten so far off this beaten path that we resort to giving ourselves and our children fiber supplements. There is a better way.

a word about fiber supplements

Please pay special attention here if your child is constipated, and your pediatrician or GI doctor has prescribed a popular fiber supplement that is marketed for constipation and GI issues in children. It contains 3 grams of dietary fiber and 3 grams of soluble fiber in two teaspoons. This is slightly less than what you'd get in two teaspoons of chia seeds, which would be closer to 3.5 grams of fiber. For many of my patients who have been suffering from long-term constipation, we gradually wean them off of fiber supplements and add natural fiber, from foods like the ones we're discussing—especially chia seeds since they're a fiber powerhouse.

oluble fiber dissolves in water and turns into a gelatinous sub-
ance, which slows the transit time of our digestion. This makes us
eel full longer and slows the absorption of sugar into our bloodstream,
which is particularly helpful for anyone with diabetes. Soluble fiber is
found in vegetables, fruits, and legumes, such as beans, lentils, and
chickpeas.

Insoluble fiber doesn't dissolve in water. It adds bulk to the stool and
helps it move through the colon. Insoluble fiber is found in dark leafy
green vegetables, green beans, celery, and carrots.

Many foods contain both soluble and insoluble fiber, especially
fruits, vegetables, and seeds. Here are some of my favorite ways for
kids to get fiber in their diets:

VEGETABLES	FRUITS	SEEDS	NUTS	LEGUMES
Asparagus	Apples	Chia	Almonds	Beans
Broccoli	Avocado	Flaxseed		Lentils
Brussels	Berries	Hemp		Peas
sprouts	Grapefruit	Psyllium seed		
Cauliflower	Oranges	husk		
Eggplant	Pears			
Onion	Prunes			
Sweet potato				
Sugar beets				
Turnips				

Our gut bacteria need plants! They provide the food for these microscopic creatures.[5] Fiber also increases species diversity, which is
protective of the gut and leads to a more resilient immune system and
lessens inflammation that can contribute to chronic illness.[6] People
with the healthiest, most diverse microbiomes consume thirty or more
different types of plants each week.[7] Don't worry, we will take this one
step at a time!

LET'S MAKE FRUITS AND VEGETABLES
YOUR PRIMARY SOURCE OF FIBER

How exciting is this . . . both fruits and vegetables are full of vitamins, minerals, and fiber. They also contain phytonutrients, which are only found in plants. Phytonutrients are the powerful anti-inflammatory and antioxidants in foods such as blueberries and dark leafy greens.

Plants have natural pigments called *flavonoids* that give them their color. Flavonoids are also antioxidants that play important roles in DNA protection, cellular repair, liver function, brain and eye health, decreasing inflammation, and preventing chronic conditions such as asthma (in kids), heart disease, cancer, obesity, and possibly diabetes.[8]

a word about legumes

Legumes (beans, lentils, and peas) can be a great source of fiber. However, they may cause gas and bloating until the GI system is in a better place. There are ways to prepare legumes (soaking them for several hours or overnight, then rinsing them before you cook them) which make them somewhat easier to digest. If you do well with things like lentils, black and red beans, mung beans, chickpeas, green peas, and lima beans, by all means incorporate these into your diet and enjoy the many GI benefits of high-fiber foods.

Generally speaking, the darker the plant, the higher the antioxidant concentration. This means that the more colorful your child's plate, the better. Most kids will eat more fruit than vegetables because they taste sweet. A great number of the patients I see on their first visits are eating only one, possibly two vegetable servings per day; sadly, some eat none at all. The recipes in section III, especially those for smoothies, will help you get a strong start.

Adding vegetables to the diet can be gradual. I don't want anything in this book to make you feel guilty or ashamed about the state of your child's health right now. We're all doing the best we can at every moment in our lives. Each time you open your mouth to eat is the opportunity for a new start.

PROTEIN

Proteins are an essential food group that serve as structural support for almost all of our systems. They make up our organs, blood vessels, muscles, bones, nails, and hair; they support the immune system and nervous system; and they facilitate the communication between all of our cells that make hormones and neurotransmitters (meaning they help with our moods, focus, the ability to fall asleep and stay asleep, and the ability to pay attention in school).

We need strong digestion to break proteins down into their basic building blocks, amino acids, so that they can be absorbed into the bloodstream. Once absorbed, amino acids are repackaged and used to make all the things I just listed above.

We often make the subject of protein a lot more complicated than it needs to be. An integrative cardiologist and friend says, "The important thing to keep in mind about protein and fat is understanding the company they keep." Let's unpack that by looking at animal proteins and fats. If animals are exposed to antibiotics and other chemicals, including fertilizers, those chemicals are absorbed by the animals and stored in their fat tissue. We can also expect the food the animals eat to impact their muscle and fat tissue. Those of you who eat wild game, such as venison, are eating meat that grazes on grass and has a higher omega-3 content. This is also why I would prefer your kids eat grass-fed beef, if you eat meat in your family. In general, it is ideal to buy meat from a local farmer or farmer's market, where you can talk to the farmer about how they grow their produce and feed their animals, or from a grocery store that carries organic beef, lamb, pork, chicken, and free-range eggs.[9,10]

Something we tend to forget is that we also get protein from foods other than meat. In many countries meat is only eaten a few times a week, or on special occasions. When they do eat meat, it is often from animals raised in a more natural setting.

Now, let's look at some plant-based protein options. These foods will retain whatever nutrients were in the soil where they were grown.

START ADDING PLANT-BASED PROTEINS

Some plant-based protein options include quinoa, soy (if your child tolerates soy), hemp, and chia seeds. One great meal example that is filling, delicious, and satisfying is the combination of rice and beans. Add a slice of avocado, chopped pepper, spinach, and herbs, and you have a great meal with protein, fat, and added vitamins from the vegetables and fruit. (Yes, avocado is a fruit!)

People frequently ask me about giving kids protein powder. I'm not a huge fan of processed protein powders for kids. Some select companies make quality protein powders, but as of the this writing, I'm still on the lookout for one that I love and enjoy the taste of. I'd much rather you put chia, hemp, or flaxseed into your child's smoothies. Two tablespoons of hemp seeds have 10 grams of protein, which is perfect for a protein boost in a yummy morning smoothie. Also, one ounce of pumpkin seeds has 5 grams of protein, not to mention a great deal of magnesium. See if you can make up your own protein drink, *au naturel*.

Given the fact that many children who have a sensitivity to dairy may also have a sensitivity to soy, when I begin walking parents through eliminating dairy from a child's diet for three weeks, we limit soy at the same time. We don't do a strict elimination, we just don't replace all the dairy they were consuming with a bunch of soy products. We do this until the child's symptoms have improved significantly. If the family wants to make fermented soy and edamame a part of the diet, we add it back in and monitor for symptoms.

A NATURAL WAY TO GET OMEGA-3 FATS, FIBER, AND PROTEIN ALL IN ONE

I will wax poetic here about chia, hemp, and flaxseed because I love them for so many reasons. When my patients eat these seeds, I'm assured that they're getting fiber, protein, and omega-3 fats.

Flaxseeds have almost 5,000 mg of omega-3 fats per 3 tablespoons (1 ounce); they're also high in fiber (8 grams per tablespoon), protein (5 grams per tablespoon), and calcium (71 mg per tablespoon).

Chia seeds have almost 5,000 mg of omega-3 fats, 11 grams of fiber, 4 grams of protein, and 177 mg of calcium per 3 tablespoons. They also contain several other minerals: phosphorus, potassium, zinc, copper, and magnesium.

Hemp seeds contain a balanced ratio of omega-6 to omega-3 and omega-9 fats. Three tablespoons contain about 5 grams of fiber and 10 grams of protein. Like chia seeds, hemp seeds contain other minerals and vitamins, including iron, potassium, zinc, magnesium, and vitamin A.

	CHIA SEEDS PER OUNCE	FLAXSEEDS PER OUNCE	HEMP SEEDS PER OUNCE	BEEF, GRASS-FED, 3 OUNCES	BEEF, GRAIN-FED, 3 OUNCES
Calories	137	150	162	213	213
Omega-3	4.9 g	6.4 g	2.8 g	0.03 g	0.2 g
Omega-6	1.6 g	1.7 g	7 g	0.23 g	0.3 g
Protein	4 g	5 g	10.3 g	21 g	21 g
Fiber	11 g	8 g	3 g	0 g	0 g
Calcium	177 mg	71.4 mg	38.9 mg	~10 mg	~10 mg

TAKEAWAYS

- We've made healthy eating more complicated than it needs to be. If we're eating foods grown from the earth or picked from a tree, or animals that live and eat in their natural setting, we'll make giant strides toward improving health.
- A good rule of thumb is this: eat close to the source. Pick fresh produce, nuts and seeds, eggs, and healthy meats, and cook them at home. Make cooking a fun family occasion. If you engage the kids and get them to help, they might eat healthier foods far more readily than you anticipate!
- Real food doesn't have an ingredient list!

rethinking dairy: science vs. marketing

IF YOU HAD TOLD me fifteen years ago that removing dairy from some children's diets could eliminate or significantly improve many of the common pediatric issues I was seeing on a daily basis, I would have told you that you were crazy. But I saw child after child improving after we removed dairy from their diet. I couldn't deny what I was seeing, but I thought it must be a coincidence, otherwise surely somebody would have taught me about this during my medical training, right?

On top of my never having heard of any dairy connection with illness during training, most of us have a deep-seated notion that dairy is critical for growing children and healthy bones. The recommendations of my own professional organization, the American Academy of Pediatrics (AAP), state that children should consume at least two to three cups daily.

My dilemma: removing dairy from a child's diet goes directly against everything I had learned—and what the AAP recommends. If I was going to recommend kids take dairy out of their diets, I had an ethical responsibility to be 100 percent confident that I could provide them with the nutrients they needed for optimal brain, bone, and cognitive development.

When I started to comb through the scientific research on bone health, I couldn't find compelling evidence that *high amounts of dairy intake alone* build healthy bones or ensure overall health in children. In fact, I found the opposite. Adequate calcium is needed for healthy bones, but is dairy the only reliable source? In this chapter I will share with you what I learned during my quest to discern where truth lies between science and marketing.

DAIRY ADVERTISERS DID THE JOB THEY WERE PAID TO DO

We discussed the role of special interest groups in our nation's dietary recommendations over the past two chapters. So my first step in discerning dairy's role in bone health was to listen to the slogan in my head, "Milk, it does a body good."

milk marketing

1980s: "Milk: It Does a Body Good." This campaign positioned milk as necessary for healthy, strong bones and to prevent osteoporosis.

1993: "Got Milk?" This campaign featured celebrities with milk mustaches, promoting milk as a healthy part of our diet. By the mid-1990s, 91 percent of adults surveyed in the US were familiar with the campaign.[3]

2004: "3-a-Day. Burn More Fat, Lose Weight." The campaign claimed that consuming three servings of milk or other dairy products daily could aid in weight loss. A 2007 lawsuit filed by the Physician's Committee for Responsible Medicine effectively shut this campaign down.[4]

2006: "Got Milk?" This campaign featured the star of the *Superman Returns* movie, Brandon Routh. The ad's caption read, "Super. That's how milk makes you feel. The calcium helps bones grow strong, so even if you're not from Krypton, you can have bones of steel."

One of the most successful marketing campaigns for dairy was "Got Milk?" It was organized in California between 1993 and 1996 as milk consumption was declining.[1] The state had $27 million to spend on generic milk advertising, and one of the television ads they ran was named one of the best campaigns by *Ad Week*. Who else was in the running? Coke, Pepsi, the Eveready Battery, and Absolut Vodka.[2]

Yes, despites its downfalls, milk is still healthier than vodka, but I am showing you this comparison because this type of advertising isn't necessarily about health. It's about selling more product. When there are significant funds and talented marketing agencies, the sky's the limit on what people can be convinced to eat, drink, or smoke. Imagine if we put that kind of organized effort and money behind ensuring our kids are eating vegetables and fruits?

NOTE WHO FUNDS THE STUDIES FOR OUR DAIRY RECOMMENDATIONS

Here is a direct quote from a scientific report about healthy beverage consumption in early childhood from key national health and national nutrition organizations, including the AAP. Note the bold font to highlighted that the study was funded by the dairy industry.

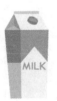

Plain cow's milk is a common, familiar beverage in US diets, and its availability, affordability, and nutrient density make it a good choice for healthy, growing children. **An analysis, funded by the dairy industry**, indicated that milk was the number one food source of nine essential nutrients for children two to eighteen years of age based on data from NHANES 2003–2006: protein, calcium, potassium, phosphorus, vitamins A, D, B_{12}, riboflavin, and niacin (as niacin equivalents).[5]

CAN CHILDREN HAVE STRONG BONES WITHOUT DAIRY?

My next research task was to verify whether science upholds the dairy advertising claims that if you drink enough milk, you can have bones of steel (metaphorically speaking). I could not find compelling evidence to back this claim. I found two of the leading physicians and researchers in nutrition at Harvard and Yale grappling with this same question: Are our recommendations based upon science or marketing?

different countries' recommendations on dairy intake

Dietary Reference Intakes for Calcium from the Institute of Medicine[10] (the guidelines we follow in the US)

- 0 to 6 months 200 mg/day
- 6 to 12 months 260 mg/day
- 1 to 3 years 700 mg/day
- 4 to 8 years 1,000 mg/day
- 9 to 18 years 1,300 mg/day
- 19 to 50 years 1,000 mg/day
- 51 to 70 years (F) 1,200 mg/day
- 51 to 70 years (M) 1,000 mg/day
- 71+ years 1,200 mg/day

United Kingdom[11]

- 1 to 3 years 350 mg/day
- 4 to 6 years 450 mg/day
- 7 to 10 years 550 mg/day
- 11 to 18 years (F) 800 mg/day
- 11 to 18 years (M) 1,000 mg/day
- 19 to 70 years 700 mg/day

Walter C. Willett, MD, of Harvard is the most-cited nutritionist internationally. He not only has been very outspoken about questioning the necessity of dairy but points out that the countries with the highest intakes of milk and calcium tend to have the highest rates of hip fracture.[6,7,8] He also points out that one reason we have such strong dairy recommendations in the US is to meet our high calcium recommendations, which are almost twice what they are in the UK and are based upon studies that were less than two weeks long. This means that they may not be indicative of what is needed over a lifetime.[9] He also talks about the importance of adequate vitamin D for bone health.

Another giant in the world of US nutrition research is David Katz, MD, MPH, of Yale, who graciously wrote the forward to this book. He points out the following:

> Most populations around the world actually consume less calcium than we do in the US, yet have fewer cases of osteoporosis. This may be due to more weight-bearing exercise elsewhere, less protein and acid in the diet, and more sun exposure—and thus higher levels of vitamin D.[12]

Please note the importance placed on vitamin D by both of these researchers. I will walk you through how to be sure your child is getting adequate amounts of vitamin D in the supplement portion of section II.

WHAT FACTORS *ARE* IMPORTANT FOR HEALTHY BONES?

We look again to Dr. Willett and his colleagues at Harvard. It turns out, there are several factors that contribute to healthy bones in addition to calcium. The number one factor is physical activity.[13,14] We must get our children off the screens and outside!

The Four Main Contributors to Bone Health[15]

1. **Weight-bearing activity.** Do whatever it is that your child loves to do, playing outside, climbing on monkey bars, any

type of ball sports, gymnastics, martial arts, or safely jumping on a mini-trampoline. All of these are good physical activities that help build strong bones.

2. **Maintaining adequate levels of vitamin D.** This means getting some sunshine in the summertime without burning the skin and adding a vitamin D supplement in the wintertime, unless you eat a lot of coldwater fish like mackerel and sardines. Vitamin D also helps the gut absorb more calcium, and it helps the kidneys hold onto more calcium (otherwise, we lose it through our urine).

3. **Eat enough calcium-rich foods** that keep our bodies from having to "borrow" calcium from bones in order to keep our heart pumping and our nerves signaling one another normally. Milk in small quantities can offer some health benefits to those who are not sensitive to it or who are not lactose intolerant. However, if you are reading this book, your child is likely suffering from some type of unchecked systemic inflammation and removing dairy may play a role in improving her health. See the list of high-calcium foods in the appendix.

4. **Eat adequate amounts of vitamin K.** Foods like dark green leafy veggies (kale and collards), broccoli, and Brussels sprouts not only contain calcium, but they are also rich in vitamin K. One serving or more of these veggies per day reduced the likelihood of breaking a hip by 30 percent in older women.[16]

THE FOUR MAIN CONTRIBUTORS TO BONE HEALTH

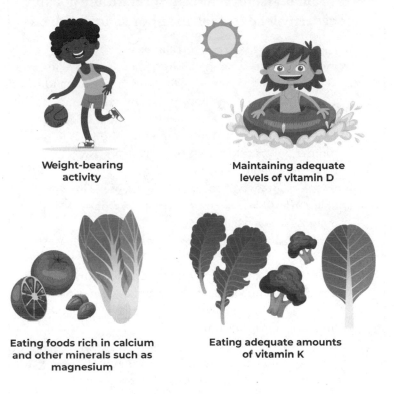

Weight-bearing activity

Maintaining adequate levels of vitamin D

Eating foods rich in calcium and other minerals such as magnesium

Eating adequate amounts of vitamin K

As I hope you understand now, in addition to the above factors, another significant way we can support your child's body in absorbing the nutrients necessary for bone growth is to decrease their overall systemic inflammation. This will enhance absorption of calcium plus all the other critical nutrients required for bone formation that often seemed to be left out of the equation. Key nutrients include magnesium, phosphorus, potassium, fluoride, manganese, copper, boron, iron, zinc, and vitamins A, B, C, and K. We need a constant and consistent supply of these nutrients to support bones and the other metabolic processes related to bone growth.[17]

MAGNESIUM, THE OFT-FORGOTTEN MINERAL

Magnesium is so often left out of the equation in conventional medicine. Magnesium works in conjunction with calcium. It is the mineral

research: high dairy and calcium intake doesn't necessarily lead to healthier bones in children

1. Calcium intake was *not* correlated with bone mineral density among children aged four to eight years, but magnesium was. Magnesium intake and absorption may be an important and relatively unrecognized factor in bone health in the US.[20] For this age group, the UK recommends 450 to 550 mg per day of calcium vs. the 1,000 mg recommended by the US.

2. Supplementation of calcium or dairy intake in children showed *no* increase or only a small increase in bone mineral density. But once supplementation was stopped, the increase did not persist.[21,22,23,24,25,26] These study results do not support the use of calcium supplementation in healthy children as a public health intervention, but cannot be extrapolated to children with medical conditions affecting bone metabolism.[27]

3. Girls and boys in early puberty who were *not* getting adequate calcium were given three additional servings of dairy per day. There was *no* effect on bone mineralization. This suggests a lower threshold for calcium intake, and amounts above that may have little additional effect on bone mineralization.

4. For teen girls, some suggest the body adapts to a lower intake of calcium (400 mg per day) by increasing the absorption. However, if intake levels fall too low, this can impact overall calcium retention and possibly bone health.[28]

5. Greater milk consumption during teenage years was *not* associated with a lower risk of hip fracture in older adults. In fact, among men, every additional glass of milk consumed per day during adolescence was associated with a 9 percent greater risk of hip fracture later in life.[29]

that makes things relax. It allows our muscles to relax and our heart to beat. It activates over three hundred different enzymes and plays a significant role in bone health.[18] If calcium is Superman, magnesium is the cape. Superman cannot fly without his cape, and calcium cannot do its job without an adequate supply of magnesium. Green leafy vegetables and pumpkin seeds are the two powerhouse foods that contain magnesium—and yes, I hear you, your children eat very little of those. They are not alone. Half of the US population does not get adequate amounts of magnesium—even though it is one of the most abundant minerals in our bodies and is extremely important to many different systems.[19] Pay close attention to the supplement portion of section II, where I give specific instructions on supplementing magnesium for those kids who need it.

As you can see, the research falls short of the dairy advertisers' claims that milk alone makes healthy bones. Since decreasing or stopping dairy for many of your children is one of our big tools for decreasing inflammation and restoring balance, we must pay close attention to all factors and all nutrients that impact bone health.

Perhaps the most complicated part of bone health is getting our kids outside away from their screens and eating more greens!

WHAT IS THE RIGHT THING FOR YOUR CHILD'S BONE HEALTH?

I lean toward Dr. Willett's review of the research regarding the high amount of calcium recommended daily. I think it may be somewhat higher than what our kids actually need. The systems of our bodies that require calcium for proper function include, our beating heart muscle, skeletal muscle (responsible for all of our movement), and the firing of our nerves. They each use calcium in concert with a host of other minerals. Why would one system (our skeletal system) be so much more dependent upon a high amount of one single mineral than all the other systems?

Then, take a look at some of our furry friends who clearly have strong and healthy bones without the obligatory two cups of milk per day (I have yet to see a racehorse or lion with a milk mustache). It seems to me, the recommendation of physical activity being the most important factor for bone health holds a lot of weight.[30]

However, we must take into consideration the limitations of each child. Some kids may be less mobile than others, some kids may be in a time of their life such as high school where they have to sit and study for longer periods of time and are not able to be as active, and some kids may live in an area where it is not safe to be outside playing. In those situations, a higher amount of calcium may be warranted.

All of this being said, I do think it is prudent to follow the recommendations for calcium intake as closely as possible while paying attention to the many other nutrients needed. This basically means eating a wide variety of fruits, vegetables, nuts, seeds, beans, proteins, and fats . . . you know the list by now! Five different studies consistently found some type of benefit to bone with increased or high intake of fruits and vegetables.[31]

In order to make implementing the calcium recommendations a little bit easier, I have created a long list of whole foods, along with their calcium content, which you can find in the appendix.

WHERE DOES THIS LEAVE US WITH THE RESEARCH ON COMMON CHILDHOOD ILLNESSES AND DAIRY?

A brilliant mind in the field of pediatrics shed some light on this topic of dairy and common childhood illnesses for me. Dr. Frank Oski in 1983 wrote a book called *Don't Drink Your Milk*. Here's what he had to say about dairy and illness:

At least 50% of all children in the United States are allergic to cow's milk, many undiagnosed. Dairy products are the leading cause of food allergy, often revealed by diarrhea, constipation, and fatigue. Many cases of asthma and sinus infections are reported to be relieved and even eliminated by cutting out dairy.[32]

Hmm . . . this follows more along the lines of what I was seeing in clinic. Eliminating dairy for a period of time, or even making it a new lifestyle change for kids with the common inflammatory illnesses, was a game changer. It often completely altered the course of the child's health and they were able to avoid further rounds of antibiotics, steroids and, more importantly, doctor visits.

I could write an entire book on dairy, and the first draft of this book had three chapters on the subject. It included all the juicy details of the following studies, which I find fascinating. However, my editor assured me the details were quite boring, and if anyone wanted to read them, they could look the studies up. So following is what used to be pages worth of information that is now simply a lovely and easy-to-view table.

I have listed the illnesses along the left-hand column and then the percentage of kids whose issue improved when dairy was removed. In the fourth column I listed some of the other potential triggers for that illness, and the fifth column contains a few of the important aspects of the study I thought would help you better understand the information. This table is by no means an exhaustive list, but it is very compelling.

Dairy's Role in Triggering Inflammation in the Following Common Childhood Illnesses

	TRIGGERS DAIRY = COW MILK PROTEIN	PERCENTAGE OF CHILDREN IN THE STUDY WHO WERE ALLERGIC OR SENSITIVE TO DAIRY	OTHER POSSIBLE INFLAMMATORY TRIGGERS NOTED IN THE STUDIES	FURTHER DETAILS ABOUT THE RESEARCH STUDY
Eczema[33,34]	Dairy	30%	Egg, Tomato, Artificial Colors, Preservatives, Gluten[35,] Staph bacteria on the skin[36]	
Chronic ear infections[37]	Dairy	38%	Wheat 33%, Egg 39%, Peanut 25%, Soy 20%, Corn 17%; Other foods that were of much lower significance: Orange, Tomato, Chicken, Apple 78% of the kids were allergic to more than 1 food on skin prick test	16-week elimination diet of the foods the children tested positive for decreased the middle ear fluid in 86% of the kids. When the food was reintroduced over 16 weeks, 94% ended up with another ear infection.
Constipation[38] (bowel movements were 1 every 3 to 15 days—YIKES!)	Dairy	68%		Within 1 week of removing cow's milk, 68% of the kids experienced a soft, non-painful bowel movement (some within 2 days). Some of the kids remained off dairy for 8 to 12 months and upon reintroduction, they all became constipated again.

	TRIGGERS DAIRY = COW MILK PROTEIN	PERCENTAGE OF CHILDREN IN THE STUDY WHO WERE ALLERGIC OR SENSITIVE TO DAIRY	OTHER POSSIBLE INFLAMMATORY TRIGGERS NOTED IN THE STUDIES.	FURTHER DETAILS ABOUT THE RESEARCH STUDY
Asthma[39]	Dairy	15%	Eggs[40] and environmental allergies—60% of kids with asthma also have environmental allergies[41]	The authors of this study concluded, "It is worth considering possible milk allergy in children with asthma, particularly when poorly controlled in spite of proper routine management."[42]
Babies: Reflux (GERD)[43,44]	Dairy	Up to 30%		Dairy allergy can mimic reflux symptoms in up to 30% of kids with reflux
Breastfed babies and colic[45]	Dairy in mom's diet	50% of breastfed babies experienced an improvement when mom eliminated cow's milk from her diet.		
iron-deficient anemia[46]	Excess cow's milk intake (more than 24 ounces per day) is a major cause of iron-deficient anemia in kids younger than 6 years of age.			

TAKEAWAYS

- It's time to reexamine the importance of dairy products for children's health in light of science. Calcium and magnesium work as a team for strong bones. The four main contributors to bone health are:
    1. Weight-bearing activity
    2. Maintaining adequate levels of vitamin D
    3. Eating adequate amounts of calcium-rich foods
    4. Eating adequate amounts of vitamin K
- Dairy has been linked to many common childhood illnesses.

CHAPTER 8

strategic supplements to support digestion

The goal of taking supplements is to help restore proper GI function, so we can optimize our body's ability to break down and absorb the nutrients from our food.

—DEB ALLEN, RPh, integrative pharmacist

THE SUPPLEMENT PORTION OF this program was created with significant contributions from the kind, gracious, and brilliant integrative pharmacist who works with me, Deborah Allen.

Deb was managing the pharmacy at a large chain store when her triplets were born. I love her story because it's not only about the triplets but also about a mother who was determined to get to the root cause of her children's ailments. I suspect that many of you will identify with her tenacity.

"I remember watching these tiny beings holding onto life in the NICU. My babies each weighed less than three pounds and could barely maintain their own body temperature, let alone digest and absorb nutrients," Deb says.

Sixteen years later, as she sits in our office over a cup of tea, I watch Deb's passion ignite when she recalls the early days of motherhood. "I could see their little nervous systems being taxed just trying to exist. They had dips in their heart and respiratory rates from being held outside of their incubators. All those biochemical pathways I had memorized in pharmacy school were playing out before me in real time."

As the triplets transitioned home and away from the monitors, Deb closely observed how they responded to things like guests, baths, eating, and sleeping. It's easy to detect stress when hooked up to a monitor and a buzzer goes off. But once the triplets were home, the signs of stress became more and more subtle (which is the case for most kids—and adults for that matter). Luckily, Deb and her husband had become keenly aware of what to look for and how to minimize external stressors. It was important that all of the babies' energy would go toward eating, digesting breast milk, and growth, instead of toward recovering from small stressors all day long. Digestion and the function of our digestive enzymes are significantly impaired by stress or the "fight-or-flight mode" of our nervous system.

Sadly, the babies were not tolerating her breast milk, which Deb had been assiduously pumping while they were in the hospital. "I was pumping enough for a small village while trying to recuperate from the C-section and lack of sleep. The huge blow came when the doctor told me I needed to stop giving them the breast milk. He said they needed to go on something that would help them gain weight and lessen their symptoms."

"The babies were colicky, fussy, and not gaining weight at the rate they needed to. I was desperate to be part of the solution. I cried as I dumped all my frozen milk and the babies were switched to a soy preemie formula. Looking back, I sometimes get so angry that the doctors didn't tell me to remove any foods from my own diet first to help them tolerate the breast milk."

Now, as the mother of teenagers, Deb has come to peace with what was done in the past while acknowledging that if she'd known then what she knows now, she would have done things differently.

Recall what you learned in chapter 1 regarding the role between genetics and our environment. Despite having nearly identical DNA and being born at the same time, the excess inflammation and prematurity in Deb's triplets manifested differently. I talked in that chapter about the variety of ways inflammation can present in children. It may be eczema or recurrent ear infections in one child and wheezing and constipation in another.

One of the kids was a restless sleeper. She was all over the bed at night and could not stop moving her legs. She also had chronic croup that required frequent steroids.

Another one suffered with eczema, recurrent ear infections, and chronic constipation. Deb followed the GI doctor's advice. "We put her on MiraLAX and gave her glycerin suppositories at one year of age. Often, we had to physically aid her to poop."

The third one also had recurrent ear infections, but her other challenges were more nervous system and development related. "She had trouble with speech articulation and fine motor skills as well as some sensory integration issues. This meant she was easily overwhelmed by loud noises or busy environments. She needed a lot of external physical pressure to calm down like big bear hugs (as many kids do). Spinning also seemed to be calming." As Deb looks back, "Understanding the significant role digestion, proper nutrient absorption, inflammation, and the nervous system play in a child's overall health was a world I didn't know existed."

Over the next three years, Deb dug into medical research. "I said to myself, 'I'm going to seek out as much as I can learn about those biochemical pathways that are not allowing them to thrive.'" She knew there had to be a food connection, so Deb went to great lengths to prepare beautiful organic meals for the children.

Stressed by her own health, and by taking care of three chronically sick children, Deb turned to acupuncture for herself. She started feeling so much better that she began bringing the kids for sessions. The acupuncturist told her about digestive enzymes and probiotics designed to aid the children's ability to decrease inflammation and to break down and absorb the fats, proteins, vitamins, and minerals from the food they were eating. This made sense to Deb, since digestion is the key to giving our bodies the nutrients they need.

Deb took an incremental approach to elimination of some key inflammatory foods. First, she started the supplements one at a time, the probiotic, Plantadophilus (Lactobacillus plantarum), and then the digestive enzymes. Next she removed dairy and then gluten. Once she felt the kids' digestion had improved (more normal bowel movements, better sleep, smoother skin), she added in fish oil. She knew enough not to add in this extra fat until their bodies were digesting foods better. Otherwise, the fish oil would go right through them, and she would have three sets of diapers containing expensive supplements that did not get absorbed by their bodies!

The kids' health didn't completely normalize overnight, but she saw big gains. She knew that if she could just remove the obstacles, the triplets' bodies would rebalance and heal. And heal, they did. She continued to focus on keeping the major inflammatory foods out of their diets (artificial dyes; refined sugar; packaged, processed foods; dairy; and gluten) and to focus on digestion with key foundational supplements.

The kids continued to do better and better. When they were four years old, she went back to work. Armed with a new understanding of nutrition, inflammation, and illness, she experienced her work in the pharmacy through a much different lens. She recalls, "I saw things that I had learned with the kids translate in the pharmacy. Patients of all ages were being ping-ponged from specialist to specialist. It became clear to me that the medical field was not looking at the bigger picture. People were being given medications that were hindering their ability to break down and absorb the nutrients from their foods."

Deb started seeing a pattern when it came to acid reflux. "The patient would get an acid blocker they were supposed to stay on for the rest of their lives. Since the body needs strong stomach acid to activate pancreatic enzymes that digest and absorb nutrients such as protein and fat, these patients don't have the natural resources to make adequate amounts of neurotransmitters or hormones and end up relying on medications to sustain them. These patients would be back to the pharmacy in six months with another prescription for depression, anxiety, sleep problems, or focus issues."

THE PHARMACEUTICAL MARCH
(Concept created by Deborah Allen, RPh)

| lowers stomach acidity | lowers GI defense | stomach unable to digest nutrients | inadequate protein supply | protein needed for neuro-transmitters | symptoms of insomnia, anxiety, depression | visit to physician and new prescription added |

I first met Deb when she came into my office to tell me about the probiotics and enzymes she had begun selling instead of managing the retail pharmacy. It wasn't long after that initial meeting that we began working together. When we began incorporating the method of supplementation to support digestion that Deb used with her children, I started to understand digestion in a whole new way.

Identifying the root of your child's inflammation and restoring their digestion are two key factors of the HKHM program. As Deb often says, "Syndromes are just a bunch of symptoms put together, but it doesn't give you the underlying reason why. All the things ending in 'itis' (colitis, arthritis) are really telling us that the patient has inflammation."

MY SUPPLEMENT MISTAKE EARLY ON

When I first started practicing integrative medicine, I did with supplements what I was trained to do with prescription medications: I used them to deal with symptoms, because I still was not always figuring out why the child wasn't absorbing iron in the first place. I was just happy to have more high-quality supplement recommendations at my fingertips. For example, if a child had iron-deficient anemia, I wasn't necessarily always advising parents to truly look at the child's diet to see if their gut was inflamed, but instead I was just prescribing a better-quality iron supplement than the one they had bought from their local pharmacy that was giving them constipation and making the child's stomach hurt.

Now when a child comes into the clinic with a vitamin or mineral deficiency, we systematically evaluate which of the five triggers of inflammation (food, environmental allergies, environmental toxins, infectious diseases, and/or stress) might be at the core of the digestion and absorption issue.

Once we identify the underlying triggers, we can begin to address the problem. We do this through a selective elimination diet, supplements, and environmental modifications—such as getting rid of an old mattress, as we did with Gary—or addressing stress by better understanding family dynamics and looking into school challenges such as a sensory issue or learning difference that may be impacting a child's emotional state. If a child is not processing information at school (or at home), they may continuously be in a state of fight or flight (stress) and their digestion will be significantly compromised. We want to arm the child and parents with tools to manage the stress and slowly begin adding supplements to restore good digestive function.

DO WE REALLY HAVE TO TAKE SUPPLEMENTS? CAN MY CHILD BE HEALTHY WITH JUST FOOD?

I've found it difficult for most children eating the standard American diet to consume what they need when starting from a place of depletion. As parents, most of you would have to drastically change the way you live as a family, by eating mainly organic fruits and vegetables (or those that you grow at home), and make almost all of your food from scratch, especially condiments and snacks. If you are able to do this, fantastic! If not, this chapter is for you.

Here's what we're dealing with and why we need supplements to jump-start our process:

- Kids don't eat enough fruits and vegetables to meet the daily recommendations: 60 percent do not eat enough fruit[1] and 93 percent do not eat enough vegetables.[2]
- Even when kids are eating adequate amounts, some research suggests that produce grown today has a lower nutrient content today than it did seventy years ago.[3]
- Kids eat a lot of fast food: 33 percent of US children and 36 percent of adults eat fast food on any given day according to

the CDC.[4,5] Fast food is highly processed, high fat, high carb, and low in nutrients.

- Kids' digestion is compromised. Our body's ability to break down and absorb nutrients from food is compromised by inflammation, illness, stress, increasing age, and prescription medications including antacids, steroids, and other anti-inflammatory medications. Sixty-six percent of the US population takes prescription medications.[6]

SUPPLEMENTATION TO HELP REESTABLISH NORMAL GI FUNCTION

When it comes to common childhood illnesses, decreasing cumulative inflammation and restoring digestion enhances the immune system, and that is what releases kids from the sick cycle. Our goal with nutrition and supplementation is to reestablish normal GI function, which includes proper stomach acid, gut motility (the movement of food from the mouth to the anus), gallbladder function, and pancreatic function. When all of these organs and systems work in concert with one another, we optimize your child's digestion and absorption of the high-quality supplements and expensive organic food you are buying them!

The path to good health is so much more than just giving a child a single nutrient in a supplement. As gut health and digestion improve, the child's body can absorb nutrients more effectively and efficiently from foods and supplements. Once we decrease or stop the supplement, ideally the child's system will continue to absorb the required vitamins and minerals from food and not be entirely dependent upon the supplement. (See the supplement portion of section II, including the long-term supplement plan.)

SUPPLEMENT INGREDIENTS

We have found supplements a necessary tool for restoring children's health, but the reality is that most supplements contain one or two ingredients that keep it shelf-stable that may not be ideal for us to ingest. However, after treating hundreds of children, I've come to ac-knowledge that supplements are a necessary part of rebalancing children's systems. The supplements we recommend here are the exact ones we use in our practice.

FOUNDATIONAL FIVE SUPPLEMENTS
(See graph in the supplement part of the program in section II for instructions on how to get these started.)

I encourage you to use the HKHM probiotic and enzyme supplements for optimal results. Once you begin the supplements, do the best you can to be consistent with them for at least three to six months. And it is very important to begin them one at a time for one week at a time. If your child has any type of reaction, good or bad, you will know what they reacted to.

1. Probiotic
2. Digestive enzyme (plant-based) *and* for those who have celiac disease or a gluten sensitivity, Dipeptidyl Peptidase IV (DPP-IV) is the enzyme that breaks down gluten
3. Omega-3 fat
4. Vitamin D
5. Multivitamin Mineral (MVM) (preferably one that is whole food based) or a whole food supplement (WFS)

TWO ADDITIONAL NUTRIENTS IMPORTANT FOR RESTORING GI FUNCTION, BONE, AND OVERALL HEALTH

1. Magnesium (kids with constipation, asthma, sleep issues, headaches, muscle cramps, ADHD, anxiety)
2. Zinc (do a two-month trial for kids who are picky eaters, or have skin issues, loose stools, or recurrent illnesses)

You will find more detailed information about each supplement in sec-tion II.

SUPPLEMENT START GUIDE

Take the foundational supplements consistently, for at least 3 to 6 months, possibly longer for more severe or chronic issues. Then see the SUPPLEMENT ROADMAP for long-term recommendations.

	WEEK 1	WEEK 2	WEEK 3	WEEK 4	WEEK 5	WEEK 6	WEEK 7
BREAKFAST	PROBIOTIC	DIGESTIVE ENZYME	OMEGA-3 FATS	VITAMIN D3	WHOLE FOOD SUPPLEMENT OR MULTIVITAMIN MINERAL	MAGNESIUM	ZINC
LUNCH							
DINNER							

PROBIOTIC - TAKE AT START OF BREAKFAST & DINNER

ENZYME - (PLANT-BASED) TAKE AT START OF BREAKFAST & DINNER

OMEGA-3 FATS - TAKE WITH DIGESTIVE ENZYME

VITAMIN D3 - TAKE IN WINTER ONLY

WHOLE FOOD SUPPLEMENT OR MULTIVITAMIN

MAGNESIUM

ZINC

PROBIOTIC - TAKE AT START OF BREAKFAST & DINNER

ENZYME - (PLANT-BASED) TAKE AT START OF BREAKFAST & DINNER

MAGNESIUM

YOUR GUT AS A GARDEN

My parents had a huge vegetable garden each summer that took up our entire backyard. We had everything from corn and tomatoes to green beans—and a dozen things in between. My siblings and I still complain about the number of hours my dad made us spend picking rocks out of the garden, which was probably twenty by thirty feet.

The land in Cleveland where we lived contained a lot of shale rock. Every spring Dad would get out the rototiller and churn up the earth, but before doing that, we kids had to go pick rocks. I don't know where they came from, but they seemed to bubble up from the depths of the earth. No matter how many rocks we picked, there were always more, as if the rocks were having babies, and it wasn't just in the spring. All summer long we were constantly picking rocks and pulling weeds.

When my Dad was satisfied with the rock situation, he would turn up the soil and very carefully fertilize it with the compost we saved all year. I even remember saving our filleted perch that we caught in Lake Erie. My Dad would dig a small hole, I would put the fish remains into the hole, and he would come behind me, plant the seed, and then put the dirt over top of it.

I liken my adventures in childhood gardening to what Deb and I are recommending for your child's GI tract. The fertilizer is our good high-fiber foods (fruits, vegetables, and other plant-based foods) along with the probiotic supplement, Plantadophilus. The rototiller is the digestive enzymes. The rototiller breaks up the dirt so the composted food can sink in and nourish the soil. If the soil is dry and hard, the fertilizer will simply sit on top of the land. Enzymes do the same thing with our food: They break the food down into smaller, more manageable molecules that the body can absorb easily.

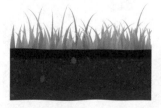

Healthy soil represents healthy gut microbiome

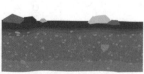

Depleted, dry soil represents unhealthy gut microbiome

Enzymes are always going into the gut and removing undigested food that creates inflammation. When inflammation in the gut is minimal, it creates a better environment for the beneficial bacteria to thrive. And it makes it more difficult for the not-so-beneficial bacteria to continue to grow (think of them as weeds). The not-so-beneficial bacteria feed off undigested food particles and the probiotic, Plant-adophilus, and digestive enzymes help us decrease the undigested food left in the gut after a meal.

Our digestion can be impaired by different variables, which is why we focus so much on optimizing digestion—and why the probiotic and digestive enzymes are such key components to our program. (See further readings for more details.)

FACTORS THAT CAN IMPAIR DIGESTION

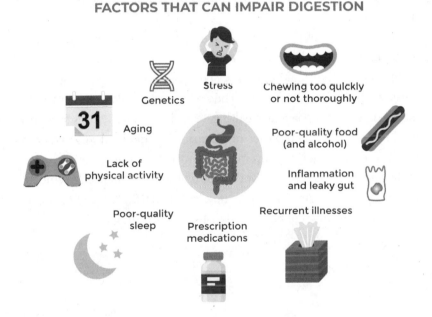

Genetics

Stress

Chewing too quickly or not thoroughly

Aging

Poor-quality food (and alcohol)

Lack of physical activity

Inflammation and leaky gut

Poor-quality sleep

Recurrent illnesses

Prescription medications

Our supplements work as a team to create a healthy gut environment for your child's system to thrive, just as my Dad created a healthy soil environment for our plants to thrive. The health of the plant is only as good as the health of the soil. Farmers even send soil samples off to check mineral content . . . calcium, phosphorus, etc.; the very same minerals we check in humans. If the soil is low in calcium, for example, the farmer will recommend crushing up eggshells into your compost. In kids, we use the supplements just as farmers do eggshells until we can get the kids eating a broader array of healthy, whole foods.

The composted food, which is the fertilizer, is our omega-3 fats, our multivitamin-mineral, our whole food supplement, our vitamin D and, for those who need it, our magnesium and zinc. It's never about one single supplement. Many medical studies will take a single nutrient (vitamin C or E or magnesium), conduct a study, and then say that nutrient is not effective against X disease. If you add a single nutrient into a system that is inflamed and not absorbing nutrients, that single nutrient will not make a difference. It's all about looking at the bigger picture and optimizing digestion, while we optimize nutrition. In order to do this, we pay close attention to digestion, physiology, and cellular health.

As you bring your child into balance, think about my dad and the rototiller. By doing the work now with your child, it makes it easier and easier to keep your child in balance because you are beginning to form a new and stronger foundation. Then when your child does get thrown off balance, getting back to health gets easier and easier. It's similar to working out: it's much easier to remain in shape by doing twenty to thirty minutes of activity several times a week vs. doing nothing for an entire year (at which point a walk around the block makes us winded!). Let's get your kids' guts into shape now, so when they face their next cold and flu season, you will be excited instead of dreading it!

Building Your Child's Health Foundation

CUMULATIVE INFLAMMATION ROADMAP

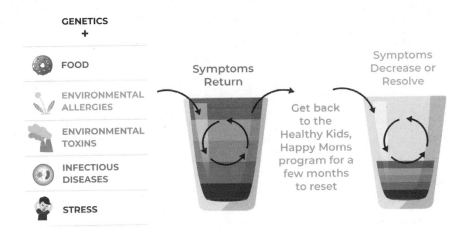

Life and Inflammation Happen
Throughout the year, there may be times where your child's symptoms return.

- **Food** - A grandparent is aging and needs extra care, so your family started eating more processed, fast foods than normal.
- **Environmental allergies** - Spring or fall allergy season arrive, or you get a cat and realize your child is allergic to the cat.
- **Environmental toxins** - You had an appliance leak and didn't know it and now you have mold growth in your home.
- **Infectious Disease** - Your child gets sick with a bad cold, the flu, or strep throat.
- **Stress** - Your child gets bullied at school, or parents separate, or a family member passes away.

Getting Back on Track

- **Food** - The family starts cooking again together at home.
- **Environmental allergies** - Wintertime comes, and the cold weather brings a reprieve from fall allergies.
- **Environmental toxins** - Mold remediation was a success and your family is no longer being exposed to those mold mycotoxins.
- **Infectious Disease** - Summertime is here, and far fewer viruses are circulating.
- **Stress** - Your child is no longer being bullied, the family has adjusted to parents being divorced, or the family has moved through the most significant stages of grief after losing a loved one.

The Many Benefits of Our Team of Supplements

SYSTEM/ORGAN	PROBIOTIC	DIGESTIVE ENZYMES	OMEGA-3 FATS	VITAMIN D3	WHOLE FOOD SUPPLEMENT/ MULTIVITAMIN MINERAL	MAGNESIUM	ZINC
Decreases inflammation	X	X	X	X	X	X	X
Gut health	X	X	X		X	X	X
Digestion and absorption of nutrients	X	X	X	X	X	X	X
Immune function	X	X	X	X	X	X	X
Cellular health		X	X	X	X	X	X
Energy production		X	X	X	X	X	X
Activates enzymes						X	X
Production of DNA					X		X
Provides antioxidants					X		
Supports sleep and mood	X	X	X	X		X	X
Supports ability to focus			X			X	X
Brain health (and in utero brain development)		X	X	X	X	X	X
Eye health (and in utero eye development)			X				X
Heart health		X	X		X	X	X
Muscle health (lessens cramps)		X	X			X	
Lung health (asthma)		X	X	X	X	X	X

SYSTEM/ ORGAN	PROBIOTIC	DIGESTIVE ENZYMES	OMEGA-3 FATS	VITAMIN D3	WHOLE FOOD SUPPLEMENT/ MULTIVITAMIN MINERAL	MAGNESIUM	ZINC
Skin health (eczema)		X	X		X	X	X
Bone health		X		X	X		X
Teeth health (gum health)	X	X		X	X		X
Hair and nail health		X	X				X
Taste buds and smell (picky eaters)							X

See the further readings section for more detailed information on supplements and their effects.

TAKEAWAYS

Supplementation helps reestablish normal GI function. Our goal with nutrition and supplementation is to reestablish normal GI function, which includes proper stomach acid, gut motility (the movement of food from the mouth to the anus), gallbladder function, and pancreatic function. When all of these organs and systems work in concert with one another, we optimize your child's digestion and absorption of food.

Supplements are a great adjunct to ensuring your child's body is getting what it needs.

The five foundational supplements include:

- Probiotics
- Digestive enzymes
- Omega-3 fats
- Vitamin D
- Multivitamin mineral or whole food supplement

Two important additional minerals:

- Magnesium (for kids with constipation, asthma, sleep issues, headaches, muscle cramps, ADHD, anxiety)
- Zinc (you can do a two-month trial for kids who are picky eaters, have skin issues, loose stools, or recurrent illnesses)

Do not start supplements all at once. Start them one at a time for a week before starting the next one.

Always talk to your child's doctor before starting any supplements.

curing
vs. healing

Kids feel what we feel, not what we say.

—Kristen Oliver, Pediatric OT, author of *The Connected Parent* and one of my dear friends

WHEN A CHILD IS in crisis mode, most mothers won't step away and focus on themselves. But when the child comes into some semblance of balance (as I hope your child will when you follow this program), you mothers get a breather. This allows you to have time to devote to your own health and mental well-being.

I've seen this shift happen many times in my practice, and I love it! I see the mom light up and once again feel connected to her life—no longer feeling like she's stranded on the desolate island that having a sick child can sometimes create.

And this is what *Healthy Kids, Happy Moms* is all about: remembering—or for some, learning for the first time—how to live from a place of peace and relaxation instead of a place of stress and anxiety. It's about balancing the two parts of our autonomic nervous system (ANS), the sympathetic nervous system (SNS, "fight or flight") with the parasympathetic nervous system (PNS, relaxation).

The ANS controls our internal organs and the processes we are aware of, such as heart rate and respiratory rate, as well as things we are not aware of, such as digestion and blood pressure.

Many of us have allowed ourselves to exist in a constant state of fight or flight, especially when we have a sick, struggling child. We

I'm including a list of specific bodily functions the SNS and PNS activate, so you can review this information and remind yourself how important it is to pay attention to how your body feels. In section II, I've also included Great Daily Practices that you and your child can do together in order to start your journey of spending more time in the relaxed state.

Sympathetic Nervous System (SNS)—Fight or Flight
- Increases heart rate
- Increases respiratory rate
- Inhibits salivary secretion in the mouth (which hinders digestion)
- Dilates our lung airways
- Releases secretion of stress hormones, epinephrine and norepinephrine
- Increases blood glucose levels
- Inhibits the activity of the stomach
- Shunts blood to our arms and legs (so we can run away from the proverbial lion in the forest)
- Shunts blood away from our brain's frontal cortex (responsible for our executive functions, such as planning, problem solving, and self-awareness)

Parasympathetic Nervous System (PNS)—Relaxation
- Lowers heart rate
- Stimulates salivary secretion in the mouth (which supports digestion)
- Constricts our lung airways
- Stimulates digestion in the stomach
- Stimulates the pancreas (which aids in digestion)
- Stimulates motility of the GI tract (which facilitates digestion and bowel movements)
- Shunts blood to our GI tract (which aids in digestion)
- Allows for better blood flow to our brain's frontal cortex

have media telling us 24/7 what's wrong with our world, and we have social media telling us how good looking and great our neighbor, cousin, or long-lost high school friend is. We have schedules that keep us constantly on the go and worry that we're doing too much or too little. We all need some daily techniques, such as breathing, yoga, meditation, prayer, and guided imagery, to activate our parasympathetic nervous systems (see Great Daily Practices at the end of section II).

Research on the mind–body connection indicates that activities such as deep breathing, meditation, and yoga can modify our ANS by activating the parasympathetic side. Activating the PNS triggers the healing response. When our system is relaxed, it's easier to improve many different illnesses in adults and in children.

When we adults live in a fight-or-flight state every day, this makes it more likely that our kids will also be in a fight-or-flight state. The predominant adult in the home resonates with kids. One of the best things we adults can do for the children around us is to keep ourselves healthy, both physically and mentally.

CASE STUDY

WILLIAM

SYMPTOMS: ORAL ULCERS, FEVERS, ASTHMA

I'd like to share the case of William, a young boy I took care of years ago. William was a former twenty-nine-week premature twin, who weighed only three pounds at birth. In addition to having asthma, he had environmental allergies and a condition called PFAPA (periodic fever, aphthous stomatitis, pharyngitis, cervical adenitis). Here is the case described by William's mother, with some of my observations added.

"We brought our son to Dr. Kilbane's office when we were not finding answers to his chronic health issues. William was seven at the time and had multiple oral ulcers daily for nearly three years, had high fevers every six weeks, and was on strong asthma medications."

William had been on many courses of antibiotics and steroids and yearly missed many days of school. He had been to four specialists (an infectious disease physician, a gastroenterologist, a dentist, and an oral surgeon). He had many invasive procedures, including a colonoscopy, endoscopy, and biopsies of the mouth ulcers.

"We were told he had everything from viruses to bad luck. Various doctors prescribed medications, bloodwork, scans, and biopsies. The final straw was when a specialist at a prestigious hospital outside of Charlotte mentioned that he could have cancer. William presented to Dr. Kilbane's office fearful of tests, dropping weight, and tired of the cyclic fevers."

"On our first visit, Dr. Kilbane spoke at length with William and me about his symptoms and pain. The next visit, it was just she and I alone, discussing William's birth to present-day issues. I told her during that visit that William is my sick child and his twin brother is my healthy one. Dr. Kilbane immediately stopped me during this conversation and asked me to recognize that I was calling him 'sick' and encouraged me to be cognizant of the words I was using. She asked that I focus on how he is healthy in between those six-week periods and how we can keep him healthy."

"After putting the two visits together, and a round of bloodwork, we finally saw a change. We started daily probiotics and fish oil and corrected his low zinc and iron levels with supplements. A fabulous pediatric occupational therapist (Cindy Utzinger, OT, who has written a phenomenal book called, *Why Is My Kid Doing That?: A Sensory Approach to Understanding Your Child*) helped us find coping mechanisms to help him with sensory issues and tools on how to bring him out of fight or flight. "

"We transformed our home so he had therapy tricks to help decrease his stress in almost every room. When his fevers spiked or he had stressful days, he would often request ear and back massages that Dr. Kilbane had taught us. When the mouth ulcers increased in number, we performed visualizations to help with the pain and facilitate the healing."

The OT also went into his classroom and helped modify the environment so his nervous system would feel more at ease and safe during the school day. The entire class benefited from the changes the OT implemented for William.

William's parents had a great relationship and worked beautifully as a team. They took a closer look at how they could reduce stress in their household. William's father took a more in-depth look at his work schedule. They had three active boys, and he traveled a great deal. During the week, mom was managing a household and raising three boys, which is extremely rewarding but also stressful and busy. They decided to make some changes, and Dad rearranged his work so he could stop traveling as much. That change significantly decreased Mom's stress. (Interestingly, Mom herself used to get significantly painful oral ulcers when she was a young nurse working in the critical care unit, a very stressful workplace.) She was then able to get back to enjoying her children, extended family, friends, and professional life as a nurse. The way this family handled this young boy's health challenges truly knocked my socks off.

"A year after that initial visit with Dr. Kilbane, we celebrated! For the first time ever, William had perfect attendance at school. He was well enough to attend a class Halloween party. He gained weight because he could eat without being in pain. He was well enough to swim an individual medley and completed it in under two minutes (and he did not need his inhaler once)! *Tears* were in my eyes as he swam, but welled more when we got home, and he wanted to call Dr. Kilbane to share the news! To quote a dear friend of yours and William's fourth-grade wax museum person, Patch Adams: 'You treat a disease you win, you lose. You treat a person you win every time, no matter what the outcome.'"

WILLIAM'S CUP OF INFLAMMATION

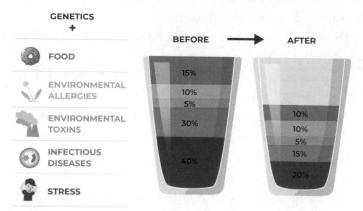

GENETICS
+

FOOD

ENVIRONMENTAL
ALLERGIES

ENVIRONMENTAL
TOXINS

INFECTIOUS
DISEASES

STRESS

BEFORE → AFTER

BEFORE:
15%
10%
5%
30%
40%

AFTER:
10%
10%
5%
15%
20%

To this day, William has remained off all daily inhalers, makes near-perfect attendance quarterly, and understands his nervous system and how to calm himself. His mother also told me he wears a permanent smile when sharing his story with others.

William graciously offered these kind words to me after our year of working together. I cry every time I read this!

> Dr. Kilbane knows medicine that helps cure you. She is very smart at finding how to make you feel better. She listens to you and wants to make your pain go away. She is very patient and wants to find all the ways that can make you feel better, not only when you are sick, but every day. I am so happy she helped me. I hope one day to cure people too!

William and his family had a profound impact on me, especially the last sentence of what he wrote: "I hope one day to cure people too." We improved his asthma significantly, but we never fully cured his oral ulcers. However, he felt significantly better, and the whole family had a shift in thinking.

I often distinguish between curing and healing. I'd say a great deal of healing occurred for William and his entire family, but he wasn't necessarily cured. We can't always cure everyone, but 99 percent of the time, we can see major healing, improvements, and shifts in how we handle situations. We can be more proactive, just as his parents were when they sought out additional care for William, but we never stopped the conventional aspect of his care either.

My role is to see the child as whole and perfect exactly as he is. I work with the family as a team, to understand the child's cellular health, physiology, biochemistry, and nervous system. I conduct a thorough history, physical exam, and lab work; I pay attention to the intangible influencers of a child's health (stress in all its many forms); and I establish a connection and rapport with the child and family.

Living more in the parasympathetic or relaxed state allows us to maintain a better semblance of peace in our inner environment. Life and people will always throw wrenches into our well-intentioned plans to keep our inner state a bastion of harmony, but this is a process, and it takes practice. It's just like riding a bike: once you learn how it feels to be calm on the inside, you can return to that state anytime, using any techniques that work for you. Mine are meditation, hot yoga, infrared sauna, alternate nasal breathing, Wim Hof method breathing followed by a cold lake plunge, going outside and walking barefoot, stand-up paddleboarding, horseback riding, jumping on a mini-trampoline, and laughing with my family, friends, and the amazing women I get to work with.

Remember to check out the Great Daily Practices at the end of section II for a list of simple daily activities that can help you and your child activate your parasympathetic nervous systems.

TAKEAWAYS

- We adults set the tone in the home.
- We help ourselves, mentally and physically, as well as our children, by spending more time in a state of relaxation vs. the stressed-out fight-or-flight state many of us have grown accustomed to.
- Much healing can happen even when an illness isn't completely cured.
- We can start to mitigate emotional and physical distress in ourselves and our children by practicing daily mindfulness techniques and deep breathing.

CHAPTER 10

preparing your mind and kitchen for the program

When the boys were young (preschool), I would pack a lunch with *three things* only. It made it simpler for me to buy/ plan/pack *and* it made it easier for them to make good food choices. If they only ate one thing in their lunch that day (which happens more than you think), I knew that the *one* thing would be healthy/nutritious.

—Lauren, my sister-in-law

REMEMBER HASAN FROM THE introduction? He was a little boy on the autism spectrum. His mother and I worked together to get him on an effective anti-inflammatory diet and on foundational supplements. The subsequent year, he was the only member of the family who went through the winter without getting the flu.

Hasan's experience made me realize I needed to put more emphasis on nutrition for all kids, not just those on the autism spectrum. Hasan inspired and motivated me to create the step-by-step guide I share in section II. In this chapter I'll give you a brief overview of the program, so you know what to expect. It should all be recognizable now that you've read the preceding nine chapters.

• • •

BEFORE STARTING THE HKHM PROGRAM

In my years of supporting families in this transition to healthier living, I have found that the beginning of the school year is an ideal time to start. That's when you are filled with clean-slate energy and carry the conviction of starting on the right foot. That said, if you're reading this book at any other time of the year, seize the moment the motivation strikes. A determined mother can make anything happen!

Also please do not begin changing your child's diet right before a major holiday or if you have several special events coming up, including birthday parties. Starting at the wrong time will only add frustration and resistance. Do not start during a particularly stressful time in your family's life either. The last thing I ever want to do is add stress to your household. Remember that stress is one of the triggers of inflammation and changing your child's diet can be stressful if not done at the right time, with the right tools.

In short, I recommend beginning the program when your energy is good, you are feeling grounded, and you have a generally positive outlook on life (which is relative if you are parenting a chronically ill child). The energy and conviction you bring to the dietary changes will set the tone for the entire family.

Implementing the HKHM program of healthy eating and drinking means paying a whole lot more attention to food than what most people are accustomed to. When you make the decision to eat more healthy foods, it means planning, planning, planning. Given the poor quality of food offered at most restaurants, this basically means eating at home most days and packing lunches for school. It also means having a cooler with you on a daily basis, especially for long car or airplane trips. You'll get used to this—I promise.

In order to cultivate the habit of food planning, begin by reviewing the coming week's activities. Identify crunch times or activities that are close together, which don't allow for meal preparation. This will help you know exactly when you need to have on-the-go food ready.

Changing your family's diet won't necessarily make you the most popular person in the household—*at first*. But soon enough, when your child and often other family members are feeling better, they will begin to help champion your efforts. Your hard work will prove to be well worth the initial lack of popularity!

PREPARING YOURSELF AND YOUR KITCHEN

Be sure to take a photograph of your child before starting the program, then once a week until you finish, so we have before and after comparisons. You can submit your photos to our closed Facebook group, Dr. Kilbane's Healthy Kids, Happy Moms Book Club, where you can also receive and give support to other parents in the group.

FIRST: Overhaul on Your Pantry and Refrigerator

Walk through your kitchen and identify the major dairy sources and the amount of packaged, processed foods your child and family are eating.

Get a big box and place everything in it that you think is suspect. This should include all dairy such as milk, cheese, string cheese, cottage cheese, cream cheese, ranch dressing, sour cream, yogurt, and ice cream. And it should include all processed foods, such as packaged foods and drinks other than water and herbal teas.

As you read labels, look for the following ingredients that represent dairy: milk, casein, whey, or lactose. Lactose-free milk is not okay, because it still contains the protein casein. As I reviewed in chapter 4, lactose is a sugar and casein is a protein. Casein is the component that typically triggers most of the inflammatory issues such as eczema, bumps on the back of the arms and cheeks, chronic runny nose, and constipation. Lactose is what creates the gas and bloating after drinking a large milkshake that even those who tolerate milk experience.

Look at the number of drinks in your kitchen. Most drinks other than water or herbal teas should have made it into the box when you were going through the pantry. Next, take a look inside the box. Let your children decide if they want to finish everything in the box before beginning this adventurous program. Or ask them if they are ready to chuck the junk food and get started! Consider motivating them by watching one of Jamie Oliver's TEDx talks about obesity, food, and sugar. See if you can entice your whole family to watch it together.

SECOND: Figure out Food Substitutions Before You Begin the Program

Review the "Remove and Replace With" lists in section II and begin considering substitution foods. You can start taste-testing some of the substitution foods before you officially begin the program.

Just to note, eggs are not dairy. So many families at one point or another ask me this question, and it always makes me chuckle. For some reason, we tend to link eggs and dairy, but they are separate food groups. I think the association may come from the farmyard. We see pictures of chickens on the farm alongside milking cows. I guess we associate the two.

At any rate, if your child does not have an egg allergy or sensitivity, and if your family is not vegan, I think it is fine for kids to have eggs. Pasteurized, free-range eggs contain good, healthy omega-3 fats, and they are also a good source of protein.

THIRD: Get a Blender for Smoothies (Or Make Do with the One You Have)

Make sure you have a working blender. Just about any blender will do. Please do not think you have to go out and spend $500 on one just to get started. For a long time, I used a Target blender my sister bought me years ago. Even after losing the lid, I held a plate on top while I blended, and it worked beautifully. I didn't get a new one until a friend came to visit and made herself a smoothie. She could not understand why I was still using that thing! She ended up sending me a Ninja after her visit, which I love and use to this day.

In my observation, the three most powerful blenders are Blendtec, Vitamix, and my parents have a KitchenAid blender that works great. These are best if you have a picky eater and need the smoothies to be very creamy. I love my Ninja because it has two individual mixing containers along with the larger one, but it's not as effective at making things super creamy. If your family has different tastebuds, you can easily make two different smoothies without too much fuss. I am not a morning person, so I put all the ingredients into the individual blender cup in the evening. Then, when I wake up, all I have to do is add water, chia, blend, and go.

FOURTH: Stock up on Storage Containers

Take inventory of your storage containers for both food and water. Ideally, move toward glass and stainless steel and away from using so much plastic.

- Do you have small containers that you can take with you on the go so you aren't too reliant on packaged snack foods?
- Do you have little containers that might hold hummus and cut-up carrots or nut butter and apples that little fingers can open and close?
- Do you have a thermos you could send to school with black beans, rice, and avocado, or soup for your child's lunch?

Avoid endocrine disrupting-chemicals (EDCs) and plastic containers. I encourage you to move away from using plastic, especially plastic that contains Bisphenol A (BPA). BPA is a chemical that has been used in creating plastics since the 1960s. It is also in the lining of most canned foods. It has long been suspected to have detrimental effects on our health, in particular on the brains, behavior, and reproductive organs of fetuses and young children. This may result in reduced fertility and an increase in some diseases, including obesity, diabetes, endometriosis, some cancers, and ADHD.[1,2,3,4]

EDCs mimic, block, or enhance the effect of various hormones in our bodies, including estrogen. It is thought to do this even at very low doses, so please pay attention to the number of plastic containers your child is eating and drinking from. Let's not only begin to form healthier habits for ourselves by purchasing reusable drink containers, but let's also be good to our planet that we are leaving for the next generation.

I try and use as little plastic as possible, and I *never* put plastic in the microwave or dishwasher so as not to expose it to high temperatures. (High temperatures cause BPA and other chemicals to leach out of the plastic.) I don't want to expose myself or my family to the possible health risks of this EDC, and I don't want to contribute more waste than necessary to our small planet. The FDA banned BPA in baby bottles and sippy cups in 2012.

I have some glass storage containers with plastic lids that snap on and off that I bought from Costco. I like these containers because in the event that I do need to heat my food, it means I am not putting plastic into the microwave. I simply take the lid off before heating it.

FIFTH: Get the Right Cooler Bags

You will need ways to keep food cool when you are on the run. Do you have small, medium, and large cooler bags available so that when you are headed to soccer, to the pool, or on a long car ride you can take everything you need and keep it cold and ready to eat?

Do you have small water bottles that your kids think are cool and they enjoy drinking from? I find sometimes kids' water bottles are so big they end up not drinking much of the water while at school. Experiment with getting a smaller bottle they can refill once or twice while at school in the drinking fountain and see if that motivates them to drink more. Consider making a chart and inviting them to place a sticker next to each bottle they drank that day.

I would love for you to also ponder the Montessori philosophy here: Don't do for your kids what they can do for themselves. Let your kids help you cut things up, and then in the morning or the night before, set their options onto the counter and let them pick what they will bring in their lunch. This will take much longer than if you do it yourself, but they may have more buy-in and may be more likely to eat it if they had something to do with packing it.

SIXTH: Review the Recipes in Section III

Three of my dear friends here in Charlotte are also amazing health coaches (Haynes, Adri, and Carolyn). They have graciously provided us with many of their most kid-friendly, dairy-free recipes to help get you started. All of these recipes are also gluten-free. I wanted to begin introducing you to meals and snacks that are more focused on fat, protein, vegetables, and fruit and less on simple carbs and grains. The goal is nutrient-dense foods that nourish and help reduce your child's overall systemic inflammation.

SEVENTH: Purchase Staples

Consider subscribing to Thrive Market; see my website for more information and a special HKHM link. It is a great membership-based online market and a good, economically friendly resource for healthier non–genetically modified food options. This is especially helpful if you live in a remote area and don't have a health food grocery store around the corner!

You will also be able to get things like chia, hemp, and flaxseed, along with coconut oil and ghee. Some of you may be new to these foods and I want you to have an easy resource. You will also be able to get organic and dairy-free friendly snacks and some of the other ingredients for the recipes in section III.

YOU CAN'T UNSEE RESULTS

This book is all about how to help your child become healthier. But my covert and ultimate goal, after your child feels better, is to help you, the parent, foster a peaceful inner landscape. Your inner state and self-compassion ripple out to everyone around you, especially your kids. Remaining keenly aware of how we impact the children around us is one of our most powerful tools. We have an awesome opportunity to lead by example. I admire you and I'm beyond grateful you chose to take this journey with me!

Now that you're walking this path, it's difficult to turn back and unlearn what you have learned. At least that has been the case for me and many of the families I work with. Once I knew what an impact food and mental state had on kids' recurrent illnesses, I could no longer simply write an antibiotic prescription and let a family walk out the door. I had to educate them about what I was learning, about a way of eating and being that could support their child's health and stop the recurrent illness cycle.

Thank you for reading and thank you for taking the time to do the hard and important things. They are not always the easy ones.

FOR ADDITIONAL BOOK RESOURCES

 Visit my website for more info: sheilakilbanecom/book

TAKEAWAYS

- First prepare your mind and your kitchen.
- Start the program when you are feeling good about yourself and life in general. Don't add stress on top of stress!
- Checklist:
    1. Pantry overhaul
    2. Explore food substitutions
    3. Working blender
    4. Storage containers
    5. Travel cooler bags
    6. Review recipes in section III
    7. Purchase staples (see Dr. Kilbane's approved packaged food list at the end of the recipes in section III)

the 7 step

healthy kids,

happy moms

program

This program walks you through the HKHM process I use in my clinic in Charlotte, North Carolina. I recommend the entire family do the program together. I have seen many parents lose weight, go off medications such as antacids, and feel a whole lot better themselves. Most importantly, this program allows your kids to participate and understand their own health.

Let's work together to decrease your child's and family's systemic inflammation, which ultimately allows the immune systems to function optimally!

PROGRAM OVERVIEW: THE 7 STEPS

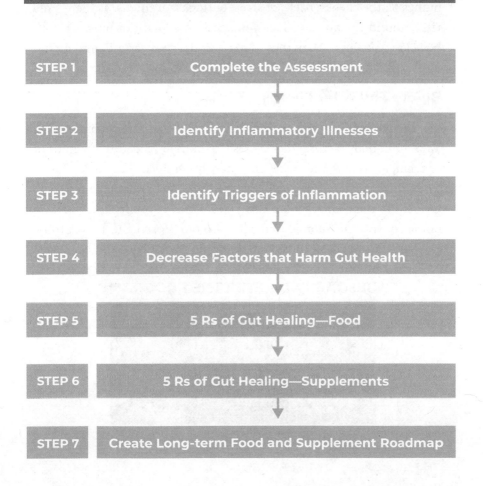

STEP 1	Complete the Assessment
STEP 2	Identify Inflammatory Illnesses
STEP 3	Identify Triggers of Inflammation
STEP 4	Decrease Factors that Harm Gut Health
STEP 5	5 Rs of Gut Healing—Food
STEP 6	5 Rs of Gut Healing—Supplements
STEP 7	Create Long-term Food and Supplement Roadmap

STEP 1

THE ASSESSMENT

The assessment is your child's current health status. Think of it as the starting point on your roadmap. We have to figure out where we are to know where we want to go. Given the pressures of parenting a child with a chronic illness, it's important to write this down instead of telling yourself you'll remember. Additionally, this tracking can be invaluable if you need further medical support.

You'll begin by taking a close look at your child's skin. First, take a good look at the complexion. Is the skin supple or dry, smooth or rough, any rashes or dark circles under the eyes? Do you feel small bumps on the cheeks, backs of arms, buttocks, or thighs? Is there a red ring around the anus or does your child complain of burning with bowel movements? All of these can be signs of excess inflammation.

Before and After Photos

Please take before photos so you have before *and* after comparisons. Take a full-body picture, then a close-up of their face, directly in front of them, as well as any rashes they may have. Record the date. Sometimes the changes occur gradually, and they can be subtle. Photos help us identify the changes more easily over time. If you feel comfortable doing so, you can submit your photo to our closed Facebook group, Dr. Kilbane's Healthy Kids, Happy Moms Book Club. You can share

BEFORE AND AFTER THE PROGRAM

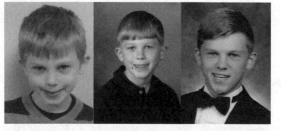

BEFORE: 2010   AFTER: 2011   FALL 2019

your story, your wins, and your setbacks and receive and give support to and from other parents in the group.

Take photos each week, from the same angles using similar lighting (possibly take them all in the same spot in your home). Take a final photo when you finish the program and include the date.

The photo example I have included shows one of my wonderful young patients who had tics so bad that he had pulled a muscle in his neck. He experienced an 80 percent improvement in his tics once we removed gluten from his diet and added some foundational supplements. He is now in college on a full scholarship and is studying engineering. How awesome is that?!

My goal is that when your child is ready to leave your home, they understand their body, which foods work best for their systems, and which supplements they may need on an ongoing basis. As they move into adulthood, I want them to have good energy, restful sleep, and a fulfilling, meaningful life.

Next, move on to the Assessment below, filling out what is pertinent to your child. If you don't write down and quantify the specific symptoms before starting the program, it can be difficult to realize how much progress you and your child are making.

STEP 2

IDENTIFY
INFLAMMATORY ILLNESSES

INFLAMMATION-LEAKY GUT-ILLNESSES

Circle the symptoms that apply to your child.

An unhealthy diet
creates a leaky gut,
causing inflammation
and illness.

A healthy diet and
supplements create a
healthy gut, keeping our
mind and body in balance.

• Headaches, trouble focusing
• Sleep disturbance, snoring, fatigue
• Mouth breathing, meltdowns
• Allergies, nasal congestion
• Recurrent ear and sinus infections

• Consistent full night's sleep
• Good focus and energy

• Clear breathing through the nose

• Asthma and wheezing
• Skin issues (eczema, bumps)

• Hydrated, healthy skin

• Bloating, gas, abdominal pain
• Food intolerances, weight gain

• Healthy gut, optimal nutrient
  absorption

• Constipation or loose stools
• Bright red ring around the anus

• Regular bowel movements

• Muscle cramps
• Early fatigue when playing
• Restless leg syndrome,
  "all over the bed"

• Muscles working well, able
  to keep up with other kids
  while playing

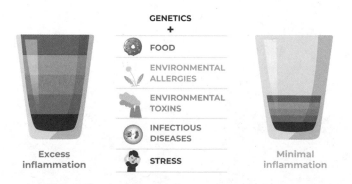

Excess
inflammation

GENETICS
+
FOOD

ENVIRONMENTAL
ALLERGIES

ENVIRONMENTAL
TOXINS

INFECTIOUS
DISEASES

STRESS

Minimal
inflammation

STEP 3

IDENTIFY TRIGGERS OF INFLAMMATION

FIVE TRIGGERS OF INFLAMMATION

Identifying the underlying triggers of inflammation helps us get to the root of your child's illness. Decreasing the exposure to these triggers helps reduce systemic inflammation, which ultimately lessens the intensity and frequency of childhood illnesses or may resolve them altogether.

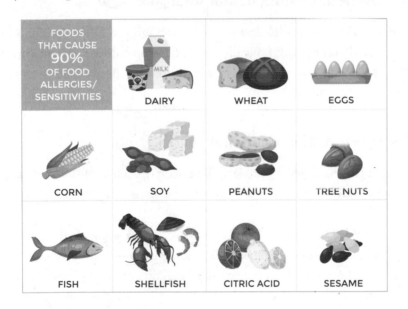

TRIGGER 1. Food

Our bodies react to foods in many different ways. Refer to the table in chapter 4, Five Ways Food Triggers Inflammation in Our Bodies for more detailed information.

- **Food Allergy.** If you suspect your child has a true IgE-mediated allergy to one of these foods, please visit your doctor or an allergist and have them tested.

- **Food Sensitivity.** Proceed through the selective elimination diet (what we will be doing in the HKHM program).
- **Celiac Disease.** See your doctor for bloodwork if you suspect this. Your child must be eating gluten for testing to be accurate.
- **Food Intolerance.** Go see your doctor right away if there is blood in the stool. This can be a sign of a food intolerance.
- **Histamine Intolerance.** Review the high-histamine foods in chapter 4 and keep a food journal (see an allergist if needed).

TRIGGER 2. Environmental Allergies

Bloodwork or skin prick test check for the IgE protein to indoor and outdoor allergens (kids typically do not develop outdoor allergies until they are about two years old; however, indoor allergies can develop before the age of two).

TRIGGER 3. Environmental Toxins

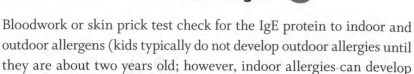

Triggers in this category are largely outside the scope of this book and to some extend, outside of our control, except for the following three.

- **Mold.** Look for visible mold or water damage (any leaking appliances or a basement that floods) at your home or your child's school. Visit my website, sheilakilbane.com/book for more information.
- **Heavy Metals.** Seek out an experienced environmental medicine or functional medicine doctor. See step 6 for resources.
- **Herbicides and Pesticides.** Eat as much as possible from your home garden, a local farmer, or organic foods (your child's body will excrete these chemicals once she stops ingesting them).

TRIGGER 4. Infectious Diseases

If your child has a current acute illness, your healthcare provider can help you determine the underlying issue. Other abnormalities may exist in the gut microbiome. For children with serious illnesses, seek out an integrative or functional medicine doctor (they may use a stool study, bloodwork, or other testing to determine underlying issues).

TRIGGER 5. Stress

- **Physical stress.** A medical doctor (sports medicine, orthopedic surgeon, ENT, primary care physician, physical therapist, chiropractor, craniosacral therapist, acupuncturist) or other professional trained in bodywork may be able to help you identify physical or anatomic stress on your child's body and give suggestions on how to address it.
- **Emotional stress.** Sometimes an undiagnosed learning difference, such as dyslexia or an auditory or sensory processing disorder, can cause the child's nervous system to be in fight-or-flight all day long at school. Seek out a psychologist or therapist (OT, PT, SLP) to help get an accurate diagnosis and support. Determine whether you have a good fit between your child and her teacher, school, or extracurricular activities. Parental stress also impacts kids. If appropriate, parents can go to counseling to increase family communication and strategies for managing stress.

ESTIMATE PERCENTAGE CONTRIBUTION OF EACH TRIGGER OF INFLAMMATION

Now that you have reviewed your child's possible triggers of inflammation, estimate what percentage you think each area might be contributing to their illness and symptoms.

If your child has current symptoms of one of the illnesses we have been discussing, they likely have some degree of excess inflammation (which means their cup runneth over).

BEFORE THE MINI-CLEANSE, ESTIMATE YOUR CHILD'S CUP OF INFLAMMATION

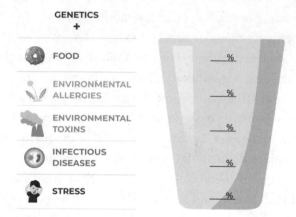

GENETICS
+

FOOD ____%

ENVIRONMENTAL ALLERGIES ____%

ENVIRONMENTAL TOXINS ____%

INFECTIOUS DISEASES ____%

STRESS ____%

STEP 4

DECREASE FACTORS
THAT HARM GUT HEALTH

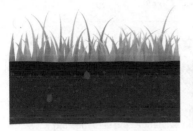 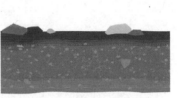

Healthy soil represents
healthy gut microbiome

Depleted, dry soil represents
unhealthy gut microbiome

Healthy soil represents a healthy gut microbiome. Depleted, dry soil represents an unhealthy gut microbiome.

CIRCLE THE FACTORS THAT MAY BE HARMING YOUR CHILD'S MICROBIOME	STEPS TO DECREASE THEIR IMPACT
Not drinking enough water	Your child should drink half their body weight in ounces.
Consuming artificial dyes and colors	Avoid foods with artificial dyes and colors
Eating produce sprayed with herbicides	Eat organic whenever possible, and when you can't, increase consumption from the EWG Clean 15 list and decrease consumption from the Dirty Dozen list. (See appendix.)
Not eating adequate fruits, vegetables, and other plant-based foods regularly (seeds, nuts, and legumes). These high-fiber foods become food for the beneficial bacteria in the gut.	Increase consumption of plant-based foods. People who eat up to thirty different plant-based foods each week, have the healthiest microbiomes. (See appendix for high-fiber foods.)
Eating at fast-food restaurants frequently	Decrease eating out by meal planning and meal prepping for the week. Involve the kids as much as possible and make it fun! (Check out the recipes in Section III.)
Taking recurrent rounds of antibiotics	Review the list of prebiotic, probiotic, and high-fiber foods in the appendix. Can you incorporate one or two of those each day into your child's diet? Consider starting a probiotic supplement.

HEALTHY GUT VS. LEAKY GUT

Leaky Gut

Unhealthy Gut Cell
Poor cell wall integrity, nutrient exchange, and cell signaling.
An unhealthy cell leads to unhealthy systems.

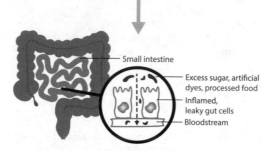

Small intestine

Excess sugar, artificial dyes, processed food

Inflamed, leaky gut cells

Bloodstream

Leaky Gut Cells of the Small Intestine
Poorly digested food creates inflammation and damages the tight junctions.
This creates leakiness between cells, allowing toxins and undigested food
particles to access the bloodstream, which leads to inflammation.

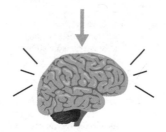

Brain & Nervous System Downstream Effects

• Emotional outbursts, frequent "meltdowns"
• Sleep issues (trouble falling asleep, staying asleep, restless leg)
• Fatigue
• Lack of focus
• Worsening behavior with constipation

HEALTHY GUT VS. LEAKY GUT

Healthy Gut

Gut Cell

Healthy cell with good fats making up the cell wall. Nutrients and cell signals are able to flow in and out of the cell easily.

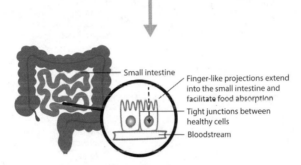

Small intestine

Finger-like projections extend into the small intestine and facilitate food absorption

Tight junctions between healthy cells

Bloodstream

Small Intestine

Nutrients absorbed effectively and efficiently. Inflammation is minimized with healthy digestion.

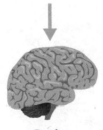

Brain

Efficient breakdown and absorption of fats and proteins help to support brain function, energy, and the ability to remain calm, focus, fall asleep, stay asleep, and much more.

Concept creation in conjunction with Deborah Allen, RPh, as an adaptation from the book *Leaky Cells, Leaky Gut, Leaky Brain*, with permission from the authors, Jess Armine, DC, and Elizma Lambert, ND.

The next two steps, 5 and 6, will guide you through the 5 Rs of gut healing

- Remove the triggers of inflammation
- Replace needed nutrients
- Reinoculate with the beneficial bacteria called probiotics
- Repair the lining of the GI tract over three to six months (about the same time it takes to heal a sprained ankle), so it no longer leaks proteins and molecules into the bloodstream to trigger inflammation
- Reintroduce foods and create your long-term roadmap for foods and supplements

STEP 5

5 Rs OF GUT HEALING USING FOOD

OVERVIEW: STEP 5 AND 6 (FOOD AND SUPPLEMENTS)

The 5 Rs of Gut Healing

1 Remove → **2** Replace → **3** Reinoculate → **4** Repair → **5** Reintroduce

MINI CLEANSE — 1 week (or more if needed!)

↓

Complete the Mini Cleanse for Kids

Complete HKHM - SYMPTOM TRACKER **before and after Mini Cleanse**

IF SYMPTOMS RESOLVE:
Add supplement and continue them for 3-6 months

IF SYMPTOMS PERSIST:
Remove dairy and start supplements

REMOVE DAIRY AND ADD SUPPLEMENTS — 6 weeks

↓

Gradually remove dairy and add supplements

Complete HKHM - SYMPTOM TRACKER **each week**

IF SYMPTOMS RESOLVE:
Remain OFF dairy and ON supplements for 3-6 months

IF SYMPTOMS PERSIST:
Remove gluten and remain OFF dairy and ON supplements

REMOVE GLUTEN — 6 weeks

↓

Gradually remove gluten, remain OFF dairy and ON supplements

Complete HKHM - SYMPTOM TRACKER **at the end of your gluten removal trial**

IF SYMPTOMS RESOLVE:
Remain OFF dairy and gluten and ON supplements for 3-6 months

IF SYMPTOMS PERSIST:
Seek additional medical support

BEFORE BEGINNING THE PROGRAM

Take it slowly. It is best to change only one thing at a time for your child whenever possible. Kids can have reactions, good or bad, to food changes and to the addition of supplements. For this reason, I have created a structured plan. Please follow the timelines and don't rush the process. You can always take more time for any of the steps if needed, but if you make changes abruptly, your child may feel worse before she feels better, and when she does feel better, we won't know which variable made the difference.

Be particularly diligent if you decide to proceed to removing dairy and gluten. If you remove them simultaneously, your child (and the adults in the household) may feel irritable, feel fatigued, and have trouble sleeping. This is why I recommend removing foods gradually and one at a time.

①Remove ⟶ ②Replace ⟶ ③Reinoculate ⟶ ④Repair ⟶ ⑤Reintroduce

This simple mnemonic, the "5 Rs" will help you remember the process we go through to heal a leaky gut. The 5 Rs happen simultaneously, and we loop back around three times for the removal process: first, to remove dyes, processed foods, and sugar; second, to start supplements and, for some of you, to remove dairy; and third, to remove gluten if needed.

THE PROCESS

The goal is to shift your child's diet to one that is organic, filled with plant-based foods, and anti-inflammatory.

The extent of food changes that you may need to make with your child depends upon your child's overall health and the severity of his symptoms.

For some of you, the Mini Cleanse for Kids may be all that is needed to get your child's system back into balance. However, after the Mini

Cleanse, if he or she is still struggling, please move on to starting supplements, removing dairy, and then possibly removing gluten.

Mini Cleanse for Kids

We clean up the basics of your child's diet. **Remove** or decrease sugary drinks, artificial dyes, refined sugar, and processed foods (snacks, meats, and fats). You can make these changes quickly, one change each day over one week. Or you could do it more slowly and make only one change per week, or even one change per month if that works better for your family.

Supplements (See Step 6)

I recommend all kids start and take the supplements for at least three to six months. If your child is still symptomatic after the Mini Cleanse for Kids, you can begin the supplements while removing dairy. If your child is no longer symptomatic after completing the Mini Cleanse, you can jump to the section on supplements and begin the *Replace*, *Reinoculate*, and *Repair*, using the supplements coupled with good nutrition.

Dairy

Remove dairy gradually over three weeks. The first week you remove it from breakfast, the second week from lunch, and the third week from dinner and snacks. At that point, your child, and hopefully the entire household, will be dairy-free and will remain dairy-free for another three to four weeks. Use the HKHM - SYMPTOM TRACKER each week to monitor changes such as easier bowel movements.

Gluten

Remove gluten if your child is still symptomatic after being dairy-free for a full three to four weeks. Remove gluten gradually the same way we removed dairy while remaining off dairy. If your child and family feel great after removing dairy, there is no need to remove gluten unless you just want to try it and see how you feel. Before removing gluten, please get tested for celiac disease if you have any suspicion that your child has celiac disease. (Refer back to chapter 4 to review the symptoms of celiac disease.)

For kids who are still symptomatic after removing gluten and dairy, please see your doctor and consider seeking out an integrative or functional medicine doctor as well (see step 6 for resources).

Repair Over Three to Six Months

If your child has persistent symptoms despite being off gluten and dairy, don't wait another six months, but go have him checked out by your doctor. If needed, seek the help of an experienced integrative or functional medicine doctor who can do further testing to identify the root cause of your child's symptoms.

If your child has experienced improvements, continue what you are doing (with nutrition and supplements) for the next three to six months (this may take more time if your child has been struggling for a long time and/or if they have been on many rounds of antibiotics). Remember, it's like we are healing a sprained ankle, except it's your child's gut that we are healing. We are also allowing time for their systemic inflammation to decrease.

Reintroduction

If and when it's time to **reintroduce** foods back into the diet, we will create a long-term food plan for your child and family.

Once most of your child's symptoms have been fully resolved or under control for three to six months, then you can begin reintroducing the foods you removed (such as dairy and gluten), but ideally, we won't reintroduce the processed foods and high-sugar foods you removed during the mini cleanse. When you add back the dairy and gluten, you do it one food at a time, for one week at a time. If symptoms return, you may need to remove that food and keep it out of their diet as a new lifestyle (or only have it on special occasions). I explain this further in the Food Roadmap in Step 7.

---

what to do if your child is currently on a medication

Be sure to continue any medication your child is on. I never stop medications until we're well into the process and have seen significant improvements in the child's symptoms. Once you see improvements, discuss the changes with your child's doctor, so she can help you decide how to potentially wean your child or stop the medication. If your child has asthma, I recommend getting a pulmonary function test with the doctor before beginning to reduce the inhaled steroid.

If you, the parent, are on medication and are making nutritional changes with your child—and I highly recommend you do—please follow the same recommendations with your medications, especially if you're on medications for high blood pressure or diabetes. If you get to the point where you begin to remove dairy and then gluten from your diet, your carbohydrate intake will decrease significantly, and you will need to monitor your blood sugar more often.

Before starting the Mini Cleanse, fill out this symptom tracker as a baseline. By filling it out weekly, you will be able to track your child's progress. Don't count on your memory—leave a paper trail.

You can also find a blank copy of the HKHM - SYMPTOM TRACKER in the appendix or on my website sheilakilbane.com/book.

healthy kids happy moms - SYMPTOM TRACKER*

We will use this tracking tool to assess your child's
symptoms and progress throughout the program.

The most important number to follow is the TOTAL at the bottom. As your child's
symptoms begin to improve, this number should decrease. If you want to share your
child's progress on the closed Facebook group - Dr. Kilbane's Healthy Kids Happy Moms
Book Club (along with before and after pictures of your child) for support and
encouragement, please do! We can do this together!

None = 0   Mild = 1 or 2   Moderate = 2 or 3   Severe = 4 or 5

Abnormal bowel movements   _____

Abdominal pain   _____

Headaches   _____

Poor sleep quality   _____

Mouth breathing or snoring   _____

Dark circles under the eyes   _____

Bumps on cheeks, arms, thighs   _____

Eczema   _____

Allergies   _____

Asthma   _____

Recurrent ear infections   _____

Recurrent sinus infections   _____

Meltdowns or mood swings   _____

TOTAL   _____   DATE _____

Stopped or decreased any prescription or over-the-counter meds?

☐ No
☐ Yes

If yes, What medication? _____

New dose? _____

Consistency with nutrition and supplements this week?

☐ 100% We were total rock stars! 😎

☐ 75% We were quite good! ✋

☐ 25% We had some other priorities but are still doing better than before the cleanse! 🤙

☐ 0% We had a full life outside of supplements and green smoothies. 😈

* This is a tool to be used solely for tracking symptoms over time. It has not been scientifically validated.

SETTING THE FOUNDATION/
MINI CLEANSE FOR KIDS

We begin by decreasing or removing certain foods while adding others in. Take one to two weeks (or longer if needed) to complete the Mini Cleanse for Kids and set your family's healthy foundation with nutrition that is ideal for the long term. Remember to fill out the HKHM - SYMPTOM TRACKER before you begin!

Note: For children who are picky eaters and/or those with a diet of highly processed foods, it is especially important to take your time and only go through the Mini Cleanse for Kids until your family adjusts to these new eating habits. Stress is a trigger of inflammation and if making food changes are going to add stress to your household, that defeats the purpose of this program. Start slowly, maybe take a month to complete each step of the Mini Cleanse. I would like this to be a fun, engaging activity you and your family do together. I have more tips for picky eaters later.

MINI CLEANSE FOR KIDS

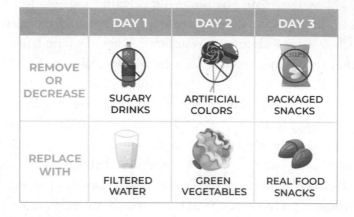

	DAY 1	DAY 2	DAY 3
REMOVE OR DECREASE	SUGARY DRINKS	ARTIFICIAL COLORS	PACKAGED SNACKS
REPLACE WITH	FILTERED WATER	GREEN VEGETABLES	REAL FOOD SNACKS

REMOVE OR DECREASE

REPLACE WITH

SUGARY DRINKS
- sodas, sport & energy drinks
- fruit juices, sweet tea

FILTERED WATER
- kids should drink half their weight in ounces (30-pound child should drink 15 ounces per day)
- adults and older kids should drink 2-3 liters per day
- herbal teas, mineral or filtered water with lime or lemon

ARTIFICIAL COLORS
- colored candies
- medications, supplements with dyes

GREEN VEGETABLES
- broccoli, okra, celery
- lettuce (butter, romaine, green leaf)
- dark green leafy vegetables (kale)

PACKAGED SNACKS
- chips
- muffins & cookies
- fish-shaped crackers

REAL FOOD SNACKS
- tree nuts, pumpkin seeds
- carrot or celery with hummus, apples or celery with SunButter or nut butter, sweet potato fries
- baked kale, crispy chickpeas, magnesium muffins

MINI CLEANSE FOR KIDS

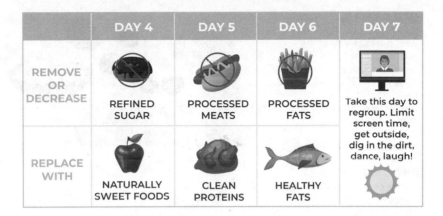

	DAY 4	DAY 5	DAY 6	DAY 7
REMOVE OR DECREASE	REFINED SUGAR	PROCESSED MEATS	PROCESSED FATS	Take this day to regroup. Limit screen time, get outside, dig in the dirt, dance, laugh!
REPLACE WITH	NATURALLY SWEET FOODS	CLEAN PROTEINS	HEALTHY FATS	

REMOVE OR DECREASE

ADDED SUGAR AND SWEETENERS
- sugary cereals, candy
- sweetened yogurts
- fruit juice concentrates
- high-fructose corn syrup, corn syrup
- artificial sweeteners

PROCESSED MEATS
- packaged lunch meats that are not organic (pepperoni, salami, bologna, turkey, ham, hot dogs, sausage, bacon)

PROCESSED FATS
- most packaged crunchy foods (chips)
- fast food & deep-fried food (onion rings, french fries, chicken fingers)

REPLACE WITH

NATURALLY SWEET FOODS
- fresh or frozen fruit (cherries, blueberries, grapes)
- carrots (baked or raw)
- smoothies
- maple syrup, honey, blackstrap molasses
- monk fruit

FLAVOR ENHANCERS
- ginger, fresh lemon, or lime juice
- natural vanilla bean (not vanilla flavoring), cacao

CLEAN PROTEINS
- wild-caught sockeye salmon
- organic baked chicken, grass-fed steak or beef burgers, wild meat (deer, buffalo, turkey, duck), organic/nitrate-free bacon or sausage
- farm-raised eggs
- energy balls, chia pudding, paleo pancakes

HEALTHY FATS
- coconut oil, olive oil
- olives, avocado, chia, hemp, and flaxseed
- cold water fish (wild-caught sockey salmon)

MEAL SUGGESTIONS

BREAKFAST
- Whole grain or gluten-free toast with nut butter
- Avocado toast
- Green smoothie
- Eggs
- Fruit
- Gluten-free oatmeal with chia, hemp, or flaxseed
- Paleo pancakes
- Energy balls

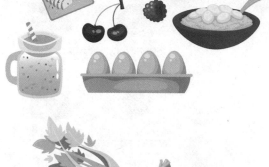

SNACKS
- Carrot or celery with hummus
- Crispy chickpeas
- Pickles, olives
- Apples or celery with nut butter
- Chia seed pudding
- Tree nuts, pumpkin seeds
- Hard boiled eggs
- Sweet potato fries
- Baked kale

CONDIMENTS / FLAVOR ENHANCERS
- Low-sugar, organic ketchup, salad dressings, sauces
- Tessemae brand
- Primal Kitchen brand
- Lime or lemon
- Coconut oil
- Olive oil
- Avocado

LUNCH / DINNER
- Jovial brand pasta
- Soup
- Sweet potato
- Baked kale
- Rice with tumeric and raisins
- Green vegetables
- Cauliflower rice

For those who eat meat:
- Wild-caught sockeye salmon
- Organic chicken or turkey (chicken salad)
- Grass-fed steak or burgers
- Wild game

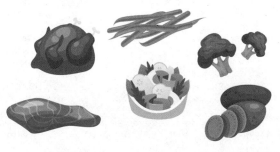

AFTER YOU COMPLETE
THE MINI CLEANSE FOR KIDS

Congratulations, you completed the mini cleanse. Before moving on, complete the HKHM - SYMPTOM TRACKER. Compare the total score to the score from before the mini cleanse.

By incorporating more plant-based, nutrient-rich foods, you have created the foundational nutrition for your long-term eating plan. Now it's time to begin removing dairy while adding supplements.

Supplements

I recommend all kids start the supplements and take them for at least three to six months. Follow the Supplement Start Guide carefully (see details in step 6).

Eliminating Dairy

If the Mini Cleanse has not resolved all of your child's symptoms of inflammation, proceed with removing dairy. During this three-week trial, it is important to avoid certain components of dairy—the proteins (casein and whey)—while still getting enough nutrients such as fat, calcium, and vitamin D from other foods to maintain healthy bones, muscles, and nerves. Remember that lactose in dairy is a sugar. It contributes to gassiness and bloating, but when it comes to eczema, constipation, and systemic inflammation, casein is the main component of milk that can drive these issues. Lactose-free milk is not a good substitute because it still contains the protein casein.

Begin by removing dairy gradually over a three-week period of time. Please follow the instructions in the table below as closely as possible. (The first week remove dairy from breakfast, the second week remove it from lunch, and the third week remove it from dinner and snacks.)

Do not remove dairy all at once or your child may feel irritable and have trouble sleeping, especially if he is drinking two to four cups of milk per day along with eating cheese, yogurt, ice cream, and pizza.

We don't want to swap out three cups of cow's milk for three cups of another type of milk. I'd prefer your child switch to water, and if needed, he or she can drink eight to ten ounces of a different type of milk (plant- or nut-based, but limit soy products). A high percentage of people who are sensitive to dairy are also sensitive to soy. No need to cut it out completely, just don't switch from sixteen ounces of cow's milk to sixteen ounces of soy milk daily. Also avoid other animal milks (such as sheep and goat) until we see how your child does off cow's milk. The goal is for your child to eat their calories from food instead of drinking them (smoothies are okay because they are blended whole foods, and fresh vegetable juices are okay as well).

If your child is generally healthy and does not suffer from the signs of inflammation we have been discussing, you don't necessarily need to remove dairy, but be sure to continue the healthy habits you implemented during the Mini Cleanse. And now you can add in the foundational supplements.

I do recommend you consider a three-week dairy-free trial at some point in time for your whole family to see if anyone feels better. But if that feels overwhelming right now, just add in the supplements! Be sure to fill out the HKHM - SYMPTOM TRACKER each week while you are adding in supplements and removing dairy.

REMOVING DAIRY

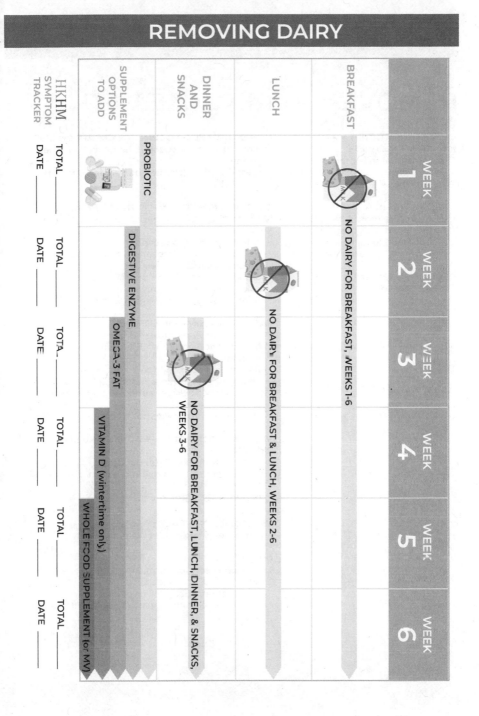

		WEEK 1	WEEK 2	WEEK 3	WEEK 4	WEEK 5	WEEK 6
BREAKFAST		NO DAIRY FOR BREAKFAST, WEEKS 1-6					
LUNCH			NO DAIRY FOR BREAKFAST & LUNCH, WEEKS 2-6				
DINNER AND SNACKS				NO DAIRY FOR BREAKFAST, LUNCH, DINNER, & SNACKS, WEEKS 3-6			
SUPPLEMENT OPTIONS TO ADD		PROBIOTIC	DIGESTIVE ENZYME	OMEGA-3 FAT	VITAMIN D (wintertime only)	WHOLE FOOD SUPPLEMENT (or MV)	
HKHM SYMPTOM TRACKER	TOTAL ___ DATE ___	TOTAL ___ DATE ___	TOTAL ___ DATE ___	TOTAL ___ DATE ___	TOTAL ___ DATE ___	TOTAL ___ DATE ___

REMOVING DAIRY

REMOVE ⟶ REPLACE WITH

COW'S MILK, YOGURT, ICE CREAM, & CHEESE
- other animal milk products (goat, sheep)
- casein and whey (the proteins in dairy products)
- lactose-free milk (it still contains the protein casein)
- carrageenan (a thickening agent found in many plant- and tree-nut-based milks)

CEREAL & COW'S MILK FOR BREAKFAST

NON-DAIRY MILK, YOGURT, ICE CREAM, CHEESE
- almond, cashew, coconut, hemp, oat, rice, pea, peanut
- grass-fed ghee (clarified butter, dairy proteins removed)

CALCIUM-RICH FOODS FOR HEALTHY BONES
(Refer to "Calcium content of various foods" in appendix)
- collard and turnip greens
- mung beans, white beans, black-eyed peas, broccoli, bok choy, kale
- oranges, dried figs, almonds, blackstrap molasses
- coldwater fish in a can with the bones
- salmon, sardines, herring, mackerel

FATS FOR BRAIN DEVELOPMENT
- avocado, olive oil, grass-fed ghee
- MCT oil (medium chain triglyceride)—coconut oil is an MCT
- tree nuts (if your child tolerates them), chickpeas, seeds (chia, hemp, flax)
- wild-caught sockeye salmon, grass-fed beef or lamb, eggs
- chicken and turkey do not have much fat

VITAMIN D FOR HEALTHY BONES AND IMMUNE SYSTEM
- 15 to 30 minutes of sun per day
- coldwater fish (tuna, salmon, sardines, mackerel, herring)
- high-quality supplement

VITAMIN K FOR HEALTHY BONES
- green leafy vegetables (kale, collards)

GREEN SMOOTHIE
- bok choy, lettuce, or microgreens
- chia, hemp, or flaxseeds
- water or non-dairy milk, coconut oil
- natural sweetener or flavor enhancer if needed

WHAT YOUR CHILD NEEDS
FOR HEALTHY BONES

Research out of Harvard suggests the following:

THE FOUR MAIN CONTRIBUTORS TO BONE HEALTH

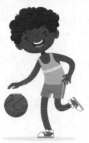

**Weight-bearing
activity**

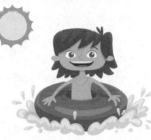

**Maintaining adequate
levels of vitamin D**

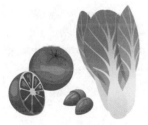

**Eating foods rich in calcium
and other minerals such as
magnesium**

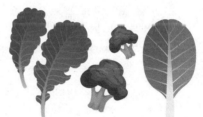

**Eating adequate amounts
of vitamin K**

removing dairy with a picky eater

Decrease the amount of cow's milk consumed by 2 ounces each week. There is no rush. Many children I see in my practice are consuming upwards of 32 ounces daily and it may take up to four months to fully wean them off of the dairy. The very gradual weaning allows us time to adjust and start to replace the calories from milk with more nutrient-dense foods. The goal is not just to switch them from 24 ounces of cow's milk to 24 ounces of non-dairy milk but rather to switch them to drinking water and eating real food. I want kids to eat their calories, not drink them (unless of course, it is a blended smoothie).

If at any moment you feel your child is not getting enough calories or you are not able to get adequate calcium into his diet, take a pause. Add more dairy back into the diet, and don't move on until his palate expands, and he will eat more foods. We are making some pretty big lifestyle changes and the goal is to set your family and child up for good habits well into the future. Take it slow and steady. Remember, stress triggers inflammation. If removing dairy is going to increase the stress in your home, hold off for now, and consider doing it at a later time.

For some children, there may be other factors to consider beyond your child just being a picky eater. If you suspect something more serious, talk to your pediatrician and consider seeing an occupational therapist or a speech therapist who specializes in picky eating. Please see my website for resources.

zinc and picky eaters

A zinc deficiency can impact taste buds. Consider starting a zinc supplement for two months to see if that helps in addition to the foundational supplements (see supplement section).

AFTER REMOVING DAIRY

Great job! What is your child's total score on the HKHM - SYMPTOM TRACKER now compared to before you removed dairy?

If your child has marked improvement off dairy, keep dairy foods out of the diet for three to six months (and possibly even make it a new lifestyle).

If your child is still symptomatic, remain off dairy and consider removing gluten, gradually, following the same steps we used to remove dairy. The first week, remove gluten from breakfast, the second week from lunch, and the third week from dinner and snacks. Remain fully off of both gluten and dairy for at least three weeks.

Fill out the HKHM - SYMPTOM TRACKER after three full weeks of being off gluten and dairy.

If you are seeing improvements, keep your child off gluten and dairy for three to six months. If there is no change at all, you may add each food back, one at a time for one week at a time. If symptoms return, remove whichever food triggered them and keep that food out of the diet for an additional three to six months.

REMOVING GLUTEN

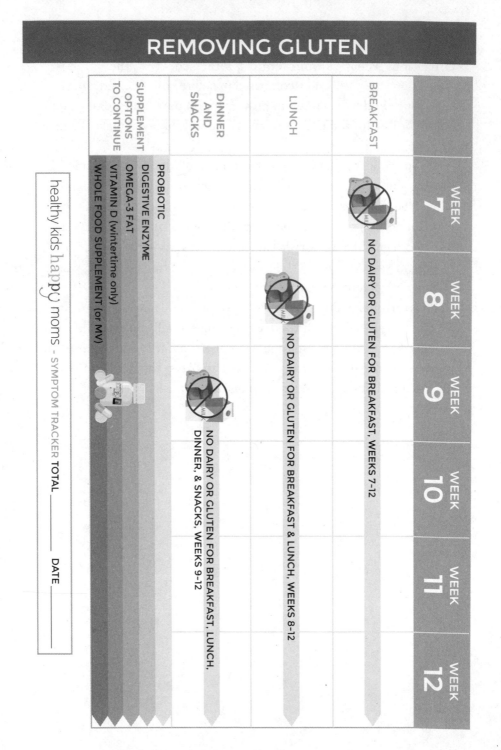

	WEEK 7	WEEK 8	WEEK 9	WEEK 10	WEEK 11	WEEK 12
BREAKFAST	NO DAIRY OR GLUTEN FOR BREAKFAST, WEEKS 7-12					
LUNCH		NO DAIRY OR GLUTEN FOR BREAKFAST & LUNCH, WEEKS 8-12				
DINNER AND SNACKS			NO DAIRY OR GLUTEN FOR BREAKFAST, LUNCH, DINNER, & SNACKS, WEEKS 9-12			
SUPPLEMENT OPTIONS TO CONTINUE	PROBIOTIC DIGESTIVE ENZYME OMEGA-3 FAT VITAMIN D (wintertime only) WHOLE FOOD SUPPLEMENT (or MV)					

healthy kids happy moms - SYMPTOM TRACKER TOTAL _____ DATE _____

REMOVING GLUTEN

REMOVE → REPLACE WITH

**WHEAT, BARLEY, AND RYE
as well as**
- spelt
- couscous
- bulgur
- semolina
- triticale
- durum flour
- kamut
- orzo
- faro
- barley malt
- brewer's yeast
- malt vinegar

QUESTIONABLE
- modified food starch
- dextrin and maltodextrin
- flavorings and extracts
- hydrolyzed vegetable protein
- imitation seafood
- creamed or thickened soups, stews, and sauces

GLUTEN-FREE GRAINS
Some grains can bother individuals with celiac disease or a gluten sensitivity. Pay attention to GI upset, skin rash, or irritability if you use these grains. Be sure the packaging says gluten-free.
- millet, teff, amaranth, sorghum, buckwheat, oats
- white or brown rice, quinoa, gluten-free pastas

GLUTEN-FREE FLOURS
- arrowroot powder
- cassava powder
- coconut flour
- legume flours (chickpea, black bean)
- tree nut flours (almond, cashew)

GLUTEN-FREE PRODUCTS
Keep these to a minimum—they are often highly processed.
- crackers
- cereals
- bread, paleo waffles, or pancakes

SNACKS
- dips (honey, mustard, yogurt, nut/seed butters, hummus, salsa, guacamole)
- smoothies (see section III, "Recipes")
- fruit bars
- jerky (only occasionally)
- farm-raised hard boiled eggs
- unsweetened non-dairy yogurts
- grain-free tortilla chips with salsa, guacamole
- rice cakes, celery, apple (with nut/seed butter)

FRUITS, VEGETABLES, NUTS, SEEDS
See Mini Cleanse

MEATS/FISH
See Mini Cleanse

STEP 6

5 Rs OF GUT HEALING USING SUPPLEMENTS

I treat supplements the same way I treat medications, because kids can have reactions good and bad to them. Therefore, I ask you to start supplements one at a time for seven days before starting the next one. Please start them in the order they are listed.

The goal is to change only one variable at a time. Pay close attention and don't make a new food change on the same day that you are adding a new supplement.

FOUNDATIONAL FIVE SUPPLEMENTS	TWO IMPORTANT ADDITIONAL NUTRIENTS FOR RESTORING GI FUNCTION AND OVERALL HEALTH
1. Probiotic	1. Magnesium
2. Digestive enzyme (plant-based)	2. Zinc
3. Omega-3 fat	
4. Vitamin D	
5. Multivitamin mineral (preferably one that is whole food based) or a whole food supplement (WFS)	

Starting Supplements

Refer to the supplement section of the appendix for supplement dosing, and refer to my website sheilakilbane.com/book for a comprehensive and up-to-date list of the specific supplements, including dosing by age, that I use for the patients in my practice. I wanted to make it easier for you to use the exact same supplements for your child that I use for my own patients and family if you would like. They are bundled and available in our online store.

Please pay close attention to how I recommend you begin supplements, especially the timing with meals.

- **Probiotics and digestive enzymes** should be **taken at the start of breakfast and dinner** because these decrease inflammation and help fully break down the food so it can be absorbed effectively and efficiently.
- **Omega-3 fats** should be given **once a day with a meal and with the digestive enzymes**. The lipase in the enzymes help break down the omega-3 fats to ensure they get absorbed.
- Start **magnesium** if your child has constipation, asthma, sleep issues, or ADHD or is a picky eater who does not eat foods rich in magnesium (see appendix).
- Start **zinc** if your child is a picky eater, has skin issues, has loose stools, or gets sick often. Only take zinc for two months, unless it is under the supervision of a healthcare provider. Zinc over time can impact copper levels.

SUPPLEMENT START GUIDE

Take the foundational supplements consistently for at least 3 to 6 months, possibly longer for more severe or chronic issues. Then see the SUPPLEMENT ROADMAP for long-term recommendations.

	WEEK 1	WEEK 2	WEEK 3	WEEK 4	WEEK 5	WEEK 6	WEEK 7
	PROBIOTIC	DIGESTIVE ENZYME	OMEGA-3 FATS	VITAMIN D3	WHOLE FOOD SUPPLEMENT OR MULTIVITAMIN MINERAL	MAGNESIUM	ZINC
BREAKFAST	PROBIOTIC - TAKE AT START OF BREAKFAST & DINNER	ENZYME - (PLANT-BASED) TAKE AT START OF BREAKFAST & DINNER	OMEGA-3 FATS - TAKE WITH DIGESTIVE ENZYME	VITAMIN D3 - TAKE IN WINTER ONLY	WHOLE FOOD SUPPLEMENT OR MULTIVITAMIN	MAGNESIUM	ZINC
LUNCH							
DINNER	PROBIOTIC - TAKE AT START OF BREAKFAST & DINNER	ENZYME - (PLANT-BASED) TAKE AT START OF BREAKFAST & DINNER				MAGNESIUM	

WEEK 1
Start Probiotic

Probiotics are live microorganisms that, when ingested, improve our health. We have hundreds of different bacteria species along our GI tracts. The research on the microbiome (the bacteria in the gut) continues to rapidly expand. What I share with you in this book may be out of date in a year from now, or even a month from now, so please keep that in mind. Our recommendations are based on current research, in addition to years of clinical experience.

The probiotic has to survive the high stomach acid to make it to the small intestine and the rest of the GI tract. The dose varies based upon the child's age, weight, and health status. We have given a dosing example for one particular probiotic supplement we have used for years in our practice. Different strains have different dosage.

We start kids off on this particular probiotic species, *Lactobacillus plantarum*, because it is gentle, is soil-based, and has many health benefits that support immune function and help us restore good GI function. It also does not contain a prebiotic such as fructooligosaccharide (FOS, a carbohydrate) or inulin (a fiber). Prebiotics are the food for the bacteria while it's in supplement form. For some people, the inulin or FOS can contribute to bloating and gassiness when beginning the supplement, which is why we start with the Plantadophilus. We find it to be well tolerated even for those with sensitive stomachs.

BENEFITS OF PROBIOTICS (PLANTADOPHILUS)
Lactobacillus plantarum strain

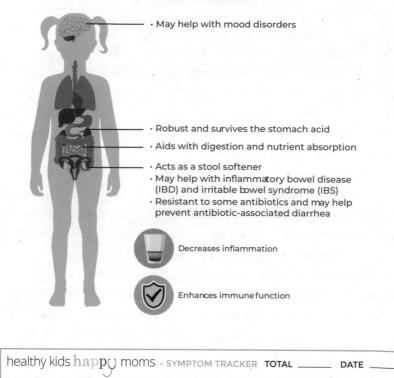

· May help with mood disorders

· Robust and survives the stomach acid

· Aids with digestion and nutrient absorption

· Acts as a stool softener
· May help with inflammatory bowel disease (IBD) and irritable bowel syndrome (IBS)
· Resistant to some antibiotics and may help prevent antibiotic-associated diarrhea

Decreases inflammation

Enhances immune function

healthy kids happy moms - SYMPTOM TRACKER **TOTAL** _____ **DATE** _____

WEEK 2
Start Digestive Enzyme

Digestive enzymes play a critical role in helping restore the GI function. They are most often a critical component in restoring a child back to good health. If you are reading this book, chances are your child has some degree of impaired digestion.

FACTORS THAT CAN IMPAIR DIGESTION

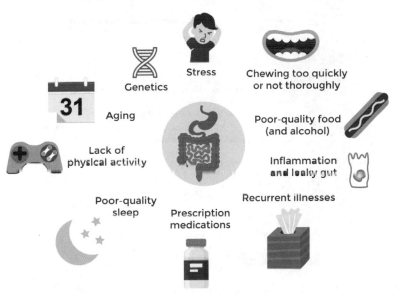

Genetics

Stress

Chewing too quickly or not thoroughly

Aging

Poor-quality food (and alcohol)

Lack of physical activity

Inflammation and leaky gut

Poor-quality sleep

Recurrent illnesses

Prescription medications

We recommend plant-based enzymes that are GMO free. They are stable even in strong stomach acid and are blended to ensure digestive support throughout the *entire* digestive system, even in those who have compromised digestion.[2] The timing and combination will help the body assimilate the food your child is eating, while supporting the microbiome and immune system, decreasing gut inflammation, and promoting gut health. For those with sensitive stomachs, we dose the enzymes mid-meal for a few weeks to avoid any stomach irritation and slowly progress to dosing them at the beginning of the meal.

Do not give your child enzymes if he has untreated eosinophilic esophagitis or an ulcer. It will irritate the damaged tissue along the esophagus and can cause pain. Also, those on prescription blood thinners should not use enzymes unless discussing this with a doctor.

Enzymes should be taken at the start of meals, along with the probiotic.

BENEFITS OF DIGESTIVE ENZYMES

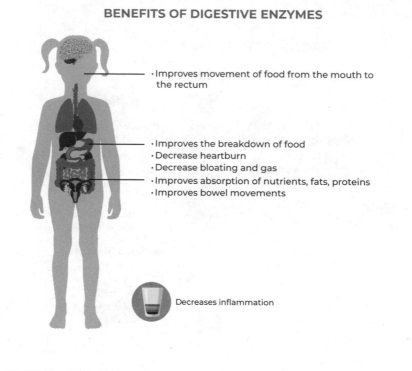

· Improves movement of food from the mouth to the rectum

· Improves the breakdown of food
· Decrease heartburn
· Decrease bloating and gas
· Improves absorption of nutrients, fats, proteins
· Improves bowel movements

Decreases inflammation

healthy kids happy moms - SYMPTOM TRACKER **TOTAL** _____ **DATE** _____

WEEK 3
Start an Omega-3 Fat

Omega-3 fats impact almost every system of our body because they make up part of our cell walls and are critical for overall health, mood, and immune system. Harvard University researchers looked at omega-3 fats and health outcomes and found that up to 96,000 deaths per year are due to omega-3 deficiency.[3]

Signs of omega-3 fat deficiency in children are increased thirst, dry hair, dry skin, keratosis pilaris (bumps on the back of the arms, cheeks, or thighs), or brittle nails. Kids with ADHD, in particular boys, have been found to be deficient in omega-3 fats.[4]

BENEFITS OF OMEGA-3 FATS

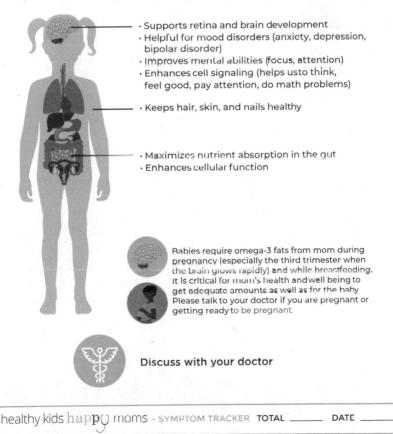

- Supports retina and brain development
- Helpful for mood disorders (anxiety, depression, bipolar disorder)
- Improves mental abilities (focus, attention)
- Enhances cell signaling (helps us to think, feel good, pay attention, do math problems)

- Keeps hair, skin, and nails healthy

- Maximizes nutrient absorption in the gut
- Enhances cellular function

Babies require omega-3 fats from mom during pregnancy (especially the third trimester when the brain grows rapidly) and while breastfeeding. It is critical for mom's health and well being to get adequate amounts as well as for the baby Please talk to your doctor if you are pregnant or getting ready to be pregnant.

Discuss with your doctor

healthy kids happy moms - SYMPTOM TRACKER **TOTAL** _____ **DATE** _____

WEEK 4
Start Vitamin D (Wintertime Only)

We have a vitamin D receptor on almost every cell of our body. It is essential to our overall health and immune system, yet one billion people worldwide suffer from a deficiency.[8] In the US, almost 50 percent of the population is vitamin D deficient.[9]

BENEFITS OF VITAMIN D

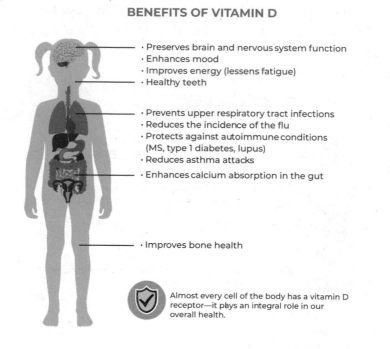

- Preserves brain and nervous system function
- Enhances mood
- Improves energy (lessens fatigue)
- Healthy teeth

- Prevents upper respiratory tract infections
- Reduces the incidence of the flu
- Protects against autoimmune conditions (MS, type 1 diabetes, lupus)
- Reduces asthma attacks

- Enhances calcium absorption in the gut

- Improves bone health

Almost every cell of the body has a vitamin D receptor—it plays an integral role in our overall health.

healthy kids *happy* moms - SYMPTOM TRACKER **TOTAL** _____ **DATE** _____

WEEK 5
Start a Whole Food Supplement
or Multivitamin Mineral

The vast majority of children in the US don't eat adequate amounts of fruits and vegetables. Most likely, your child falls short somewhere as well and would benefit from a whole food supplement or multivitamin mineral.

BENEFITS OF A WHOLE FOOD SUPPLEMENT

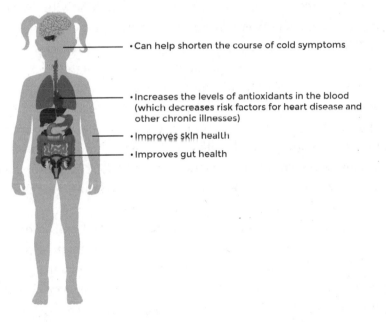

- Can help shorten the course of cold symptoms
- Increases the levels of antioxidants in the blood (which decreases risk factors for heart disease and other chronic illnesses)
- Improves skin health
- Improves gut health

healthy kids happy moms - SYMPTOM TRACKER TOTAL _____ DATE _____

WEEK 6
Start Magnesium If Needed

Half of the US population does not get adequate amounts of magnesium. It is one of the most abundant minerals in our bodies and is extremely important to many different systems.[10] I suspect most of your children would benefit from a magnesium supplement. Most of the patients in my practice are on magnesium.

Signs of depletion include loss of appetite, nausea, fatigue, constipation, asthma, trouble sleeping, headaches, muscle cramps, fatigue, high blood pressure, heart palpitations (only if working with a cardiologist), ADHD, and anxiety. More severe signs can be numbness and tingling in the limbs, seizures, and more serious heart issues.

The magnesium that you might purchase in a drug store or grocery store is *not* what I would recommend, unless you just need it to get your bowels moving over the course of a few days to a couple of weeks. Typically, drug store supplements are in the form of magnesium citrate or magnesium oxide (think milk of magnesia). They remain in the GI tract and will help with constipation, but they don't get absorbed into the bloodstream. They may irritate the GI tract lining if taken over a longer period of time.

The magnesium I use in my practice is gentle and well absorbed (it has some magnesium citrate in addition to magnesium glycinate). Therefore, it helps with constipation and supports our many bodily processes that require magnesium. Some other gentle forms of magnesium include magnesium malate and magnesium L-Threonate. Refer to my website sheilakilbane.com/book for specific brands.

Constipation (Magnesium + Fiber)

Magnesium and fiber are two critical factors to resolving constipation. Fiber adds substance or bulk to your stool, promoting regular bowel movements. Many children's fiber supplements contain added sugar, corn oil, and other ingredients I would rather not have your child ingesting. There are many supplements on the market for fiber, but I'd like you to consider increasing your child's fiber intake through food instead of using a supplement. One to two teaspoons of chia, hemp, or flaxseed mixed into a smoothie or incorporated into the diet daily are a great way to increase fiber.

BENEFITS OF MAGNESIUM

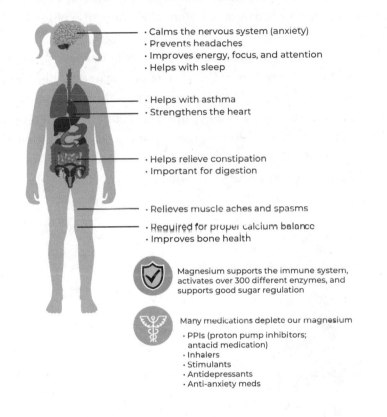

- Calms the nervous system (anxiety)
- Prevents headaches
- Improves energy, focus, and attention
- Helps with sleep

- Helps with asthma
- Strengthens the heart

- Helps relieve constipation
- Important for digestion

- Relieves muscle aches and spasms
- Required for proper calcium balance
- Improves bone health

Magnesium supports the immune system, activates over 300 different enzymes, and supports good sugar regulation

Many medications deplete our magnesium

- PPIs (proton pump inhibitors; antacid medication)
- Inhalers
- Stimulants
- Antidepressants
- Anti-anxiety meds

healthy kids happy moms   SYMPTOM TRACKER   **TOTAL** _____   **DATE** _____

WEEK 7
Start Zinc If Needed

Severe zinc deficiency is rare in developed countries, but even mild to moderate deficiencies can significantly impact the immune system.

Zinc is a trace mineral, which means we only need small amounts for good health. Our bodies do not store zinc. We must consume adequate amounts regularly.

Blood levels checked on standard labs may not always be a good reflection of the true picture of the amount of zinc in the cells. Identifying if your child is eating adequate amounts daily and if he has any of the indicators of a zinc deficiency may be a better barometer. Older infants (seven- to twelve-month range) who are solely breastfed are also at increased risk if they are not eating foods rich in zinc. Formula is fortified, so formula-fed babies should have adequate amounts.

BENEFITS OF ZINC

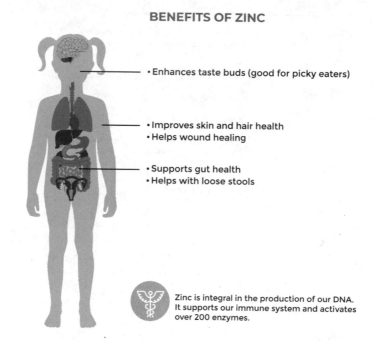

• Enhances taste buds (good for picky eaters)

• Improves skin and hair health
• Helps wound healing

• Supports gut health
• Helps with loose stools

Zinc is integral in the production of our DNA. It supports our immune system and activates over 200 enzymes.

healthy kids happy moms - SYMPTOM TRACKER   TOTAL _____ DATE _____

You can do a two-month trial of zinc if your child has any of the following: picky eating, poor appetite, poor growth, developmental delays, cognitive difficulties, recurrent illnesses (kids who have been on many rounds of antibiotics), loose stools or diarrhea, hair loss, delayed puberty, eye or skin issues such as eczema, or recurrent rashes.[11,12,13,14,15]

HOW LONG SHOULD YOUR CHILD TAKE THE SUPPLEMENTS?

My goal is for your child to take the foundational supplements consistently for the next three to six months. If your child has been on many rounds of antibiotics or steroids and has been in the cycle of recurrent illnesses for several years, it may take up to a year or more for their systemic inflammation to improve. But you should see small, incremental improvements as you consistently keep up with improved nutrition and the supplements.

SEEKING OUT ADDITIONAL MEDICAL SUPPORT
An Integrative or Functional Medicine Doctor

If your child is still symptomatic after removing gluten and dairy (and possibly any other food you felt your child might be reacting to such as eggs), seek out additional medical support.

It is possible that something else in addition to or other than food may be triggering your child's inflammation and symptoms. I don't recommend you remove any further food groups from your child's diet after removing dairy and gluten (with the exception of eggs and high-histamine foods for kids with eczema) without the guidance of a doctor and registered dietician. When we eliminate major food groups, we start to decrease fiber, fats, proteins, and other nutrients, and we want to make sure your child is getting what he or she needs.

Review the five triggers of inflammation and consider seeking the help of an integrative or conventional medical doctor. We always have to keep in mind that a more serious underlying illness may be contributing to your child's symptoms. More extensive testing may be warranted. An autoimmune condition such as inflammatory bowel disease, thyroid disease or lupus, or significant gut dysbiosis (small intestine bacterial overgrowth (SIBO), mold illness, or some type of underlying genetic abnormality may be present.

My office is open to new patients. You are welcome to reach out and inquire about becoming a patient in our practice.

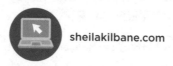 sheilakilbane.com

Or find a practitioner near you:

Integrative Medical Doctors

Website: The University of Arizona Andrew Weil Center for Integrative Medicine—Find an Integrative Health and Medical Professional

Functional Medicine Doctors

Website: The Institute for Functional Medicine—Find a Practitioner

STEP 7

CREATE THE LONG-TERM FOOD AND SUPPLEMENT ROADMAP FOR YOUR CHILD

REINTRODUCING FOODS

Whether, When, and How to Reintroduce Dairy and Gluten Back Into the Diet

In my experience, it takes at least three to six months, sometimes longer, to improve a child's leaky gut. Although symptoms often begin improving within the first one to four weeks, the more serious your child's symptoms were initially, the longer you may need to be diligent with the nutrition and supplements. It can take longer for some children (especially kids with asthma and those who have been on many rounds of antibiotics for ear or sinus infections) to bring their systemic inflammation under control and see significant and long-lasting changes.

If, after three to six months, your child's symptoms are significantly improved, you may proceed with adding dairy and/or gluten back into the diet. Add them back one at a time, for one week at a time. Be on the lookout for worsening skin rash, rosy cheeks, abdominal pain, abnormal stools (loose or hard), red ring around the anus, trouble sleeping, or an increase in irritability, moodiness, or behavior challenges.

Sometimes it is upon reintroducing the foods that we figure out the child is reacting to it. If you see symptoms worsen, remove that food for another three to six months. For some kids, if the food triggers symptoms each time you reintroduce it, you may need to keep that food out of their diet as a new lifestyle.

Some kids may only have an issue with gluten and not dairy or vice versa, or eggs may be their only problem food. As your child's health continues to improve, you can continue to reintroduce a food and watch for reactions.

Once you figure out the nutrition that works best for your child (which foods they need to continue avoiding and which healthy foods they can eat), follow the Food Roadmap.

If your child's symptoms improve dramatically upon removal of gluten and/or dairy, I would strongly recommend you consider remaining off the foods your child reacted to as a lifestyle. If it has been difficult for your family to maintain the dairy- and/or gluten-free status, you can reintroduce the food groups one at a time, for one week at a time, as described above and see how they do.

We can usually get to a point where the kids can enjoy the food intermittently, without having a big flare of the symptoms they had when you started the program. Most kids eat far too much dairy and gluten regularly. If you can keep your child's consumption down to only occasionally and in small amounts, such as birthday parties or special occasions, that is ideal.

THE FOOD ROADMAP

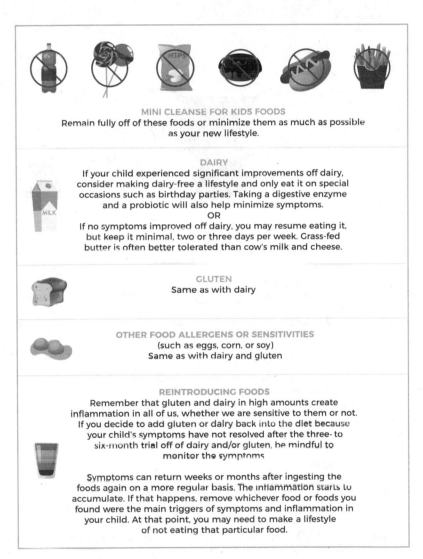

MINI CLEANSE FOR KIDS FOODS
Remain fully off of these foods or minimize them as much as possible as your new lifestyle.

DAIRY
If your child experienced significant improvements off dairy, consider making dairy-free a lifestyle and only eat it on special occasions such as birthday parties. Taking a digestive enzyme and a probiotic will also help minimize symptoms.

OR

If no symptoms improved off dairy, you may resume eating it, but keep it minimal, two or three days per week. Grass-fed butter is often better tolerated than cow's milk and cheese.

GLUTEN
Same as with dairy

OTHER FOOD ALLERGENS OR SENSITIVITIES
(such as eggs, corn, or soy)
Same as with dairy and gluten

REINTRODUCING FOODS
Remember that gluten and dairy in high amounts create inflammation in all of us, whether we are sensitive to them or not. If you decide to add gluten or dairy back into the diet because your child's symptoms have not resolved after the three- to six-month trial off of dairy and/or gluten, be mindful to monitor the symptoms

Symptoms can return weeks or months after ingesting the foods again on a more regular basis. The inflammation starts to accumulate. If that happens, remove whichever food or foods you found were the main triggers of symptoms and inflammation in your child. At that point, you may need to make a lifestyle of not eating that particular food.

CUMULATIVE INFLAMMATION ROADMAP

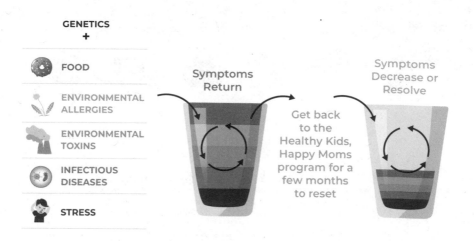

GENETICS
+

FOOD

ENVIRONMENTAL ALLERGIES

ENVIRONMENTAL TOXINS

INFECTIOUS DISEASES

STRESS

Symptoms Return

Get back to the Healthy Kids, Happy Moms program for a few months to reset

Symptoms Decrease or Resolve

Life and Inflammation Happen
Throughout the year, there may be times where your child's symptoms return.

- **Food** - A grandparent is aging and needs extra care, so your family started eating more processed, fast foods than normal.
- **Environmental allergies** - Spring or fall allergy season arrive, or you get a cat and realize your child is allergic to the cat.
- **Environmental toxins** - You had an appliance leak and didn't know it and now you have mold growth in your home.
- **Infectious Disease** - Your child gets sick with a bad cold, the flu, or strep throat.
- **Stress** - Your child gets bullied at school, or parents separate, or a family member passes away.

Getting Back on Track

- **Food** - The family starts cooking again together at home.
- **Environmental allergies** - Wintertime comes, and the cold weather brings a reprieve from fall allergies.
- **Environmental toxins** - Mold remediation was a success and your family is no longer being exposed to those mold mycotoxins.
- **Infectious Disease** - Summertime is here, and far fewer viruses are circulating.
- **Stress** - Your child is no longer being bullied, the family has adjusted to parents being divorced, or the family has moved through the most significant stages of grief after losing a loved one.

SUPPLEMENT ROADMAP

	WINTER	SPRING	SUMMER	FALL
PROBIOTIC	TAKE DURING COLD WEATHER MONTHS			TAKE DURING COLD WEATHER MONTHS
DIGESTIVE ENZYME	TAKE AS NEEDED FOR DIGESTIVE ISSUES			
OMEGA-3 FATS	TAKE YEAR ROUND IF YOUR CHILD IS NOT EATING OMEGA-3 RICH FOODS (SEE APPENDIX) OR IF HE/SHE HAS ECZEMA, RECURRENT ILLNESSES, ASTHMA, ALLERGIES, CONSTIPATION, ADHD, OR ANXIETY			
VITAMIN D3	TAKE DURING COLD WEATHER MONTHS			TAKE DURING COLD WEATHER MONTHS
WHOLE FOOD SUPPLEMENT OR MULTIVITAMIN MINERAL	TAKE YEAR ROUND			
MAGNESIUM	TAKE YEAR ROUND IF YOUR CHILD IS NOT EATING MAGNESIUM RICH FOODS (SEE APPENDIX) OR IF HE/SHE HAS CONSTIPATION, ASTHMA, SLEEP ISSUES, HEADACHES, MUSCLE CRAMPS, ADHD, OR ANXIETY			
ZINC	A TRIAL OF ZINC MAY BE BENEFICIAL FOR KIDS NOT EATING ZINC RICH FOODS (SEE APPENDIX) OR FOR PICKY EATERS ECZEMA, LOOSE STOOLS, OR RECURRENT ILLNESSES. DO NOT TAKE LONGER THAN 2 MONTHS UNLESS BEING FOLLOWED BY YOUR DOCTOR BECAUSE ZINC CAN IMPACT COPPER LEVELS			

BEING PROACTIVE FOR COLD AND FLU SEASON

Consider implementing as many parts of the HKHM program as possible during cold and flu season each year. See my website for additional supplements to support the immune system.

IMMUNE SUPPORT FOR COLD AND FLU SEASON

On my website, you can access information about additional immune supportive supplements for cold and flu season.

 sheilakilbane.com/home

What we know about the body's ability to withstand viruses and bacteria is that the better off we are from a nutritional and gut health standpoint, the more likely we are to avoid a serious course of illness, whether it's the common cold, the flu virus, or gastroenteritis (diarrhea and vomiting). Nutrition and supplements have not been shown to be treatments for these illnesses, but well-nourished children have time and time again shown to be less prone to recurrent illnesses.[16,17,18]

This goes back to the case I shared in the introduction. My young patient Hasan who had autism. He was on a healthy, anti-inflammatory diet, along with the foundational supplements. When the flu moved rapidly through his household, he was the only one who did not get sick. Yes, this is just one case scenario, but I have seen this play out hundreds of times with my patients. Once we give the immune system what it needs to do its job, it works great. I encourage you not to continuously say out loud, Johnny has a weak immune system, but rather, Johnny has a strong immune system because we are now giving him the food and supplements that are right for his body.

ADDITIONAL TIPS FOR
A SUCCESSFUL PROGRAM

Great Daily Practices

Great Daily Practices (GDPs) to start (or continue if you are already doing them):

Drink Plenty of Water.

5 to 8 years	5 glasses (1 liter)
9 to 12 years	7 glasses (1½ liters)
13 years+	8 to 10 glasses (2 liters)

Get Outside Every Day, Walk in the Woods, and Go Barefoot When You Can! If possible, run around barefoot for fifteen to thirty minutes. There is a large body of research on the positive effects of being outside barefoot. It triggers the relaxation side of our nervous system (the parasympathetic nervous system).

Refer to the blog on my website for the health benefits of being barefoot.

Get Adequate Sun Exposure. Fifteen to thirty minutes without sunscreen but without burning. Our body synthesizes vitamin D through the skin.

Play in the Dirt. A great way to reinoculate your child's gut bacteria is to have her play in the dirt! My friend Maya Shetreat, MD, wrote a book called *The Dirt Cure*, which outlines the many reasons getting back to nature is one of the best things we can do for ourselves and our children.

Minimize Screen Time. Ideally, this would be less than one hour per day, and if possible, unplug the TV during the school week.

Breathe Deeply. Sit and breathe deeply with your child for two minutes once a day. Actually, sit down and set a timer, and just inhale and exhale. You can look up my YouTube video, *Alternate nasal breathing in children for more focus and for calming*, where I teach kids how to do alternate nasal breathing.

Gratitude Journal. Write down three things every morning and every evening for which you are grateful. How fun would this be if you and your child did this together each evening or each morning? Please give yourself some kudos about what an *incredible* parent you are. Write down what makes you uniquely qualified to be the parent you are to your child. Please keep up the positive self-talk for yourself so you can model that for your child. We must drown out the all-too-familiar negative voice that many of us have in our heads! Consider getting a copy of *The Five-Minute Journal* to jump-start your new habit.

Set Your Daily Intention and Your State of Being. I have developed a system for my mornings. At the suggestion of my friend Kristen Oliver, author of *The Connected Parent*, I first choose how I will feel each day (getting into the *flow state or state of gratitude*), and then I write down three things I am grateful for and the top three things I want to accomplish that day. Kristen, as well as many holy books, suggests that our emotional state is the most important thing. Circumstances around us will always fluctuate. Someone or something in our lives will always fail to live up to our expectations. If we can choose our state, it allows us to remove the expectations we place on others (especially our children and significant others) and liberates them from having to live up to these expectations. The more we can get into the flow state, the more often we will be the drivers of our emotions. There are many ways to get into this state, and it does not have to take a long time. A few minutes each morning is better than not at all! The flow state might be entered through a few minutes of silence or deep breathing, prayer, reading a holy book, reading inspirational quotes, meditation, yoga, rigorous physical activity, or even walking slowly outside.

Switch to More Natural Hair and Body Care Products. Many beauty products (soaps, shampoos, lotions, makeup, toothpaste, mouthwash, deodorant) have harmful ingredients (parabens and phthalates plus many others). Please look up what you are using on the website of the Environmental Working Group (EWG Skin Deep® Cosmetics Database) and start switching to more natural products. Also avoid products with artificial dyes.

Switch to More Natural Cleaning Products. Many cleaning products have powerful and harmful ingredients. Consider switching to vinegar and water to clean hardwood floors and windows, and baking soda and water to clean sinks, toilets, and bathtubs.

SECTION III

the

recipes

smoothies and cashew milk

GETTING STARTED WITH SMOOTHIES

Smoothies give us the perfect kickstart to this process of restoring health. Even if you are not going to remove dairy 100 percent from your child's diet, I would still recommend removing it from breakfast if possible. Smoothies are a great way to do this.

I can hear you thinking right now, "My child is not going to drink a green smoothie!" Continue reading for some tips and tricks to get your child interested in smoothies.

SIMPLE SMOOTHIE TIPS

Let's take a step back and talk about how you might approach this with your not-so-eager child. Part of the fun of this program is being in the kitchen with your child. It may take some creative mixing to find a nutrient-dense smoothie with the taste and texture that he will drink.

What if you make this a great kitchen and food adventure with your child? What would get him interested? Is it color, concoction, different flavors, or her participation as mom and dad prepare meals? Play with this to see what excites your child.

LIQUID FOR SMOOTHIES

The liquid base of these smoothies should ideally be water. If you can, try not to use commercial juice products or cow's milk yogurt because of the sugar. Juices bought in the store, even if they are organic, are predominantly sugar. Freshly extracted vegetable juices are an entirely different ball game and are extremely healthful.

Unsweetened non-dairy milk or non-dairy yogurts are another option if your child and family are craving a creamier smoothie. However, the sweetened non-dairy milks and yogurts may contain a significant amount of sugar, so my first preference will always be water.

PICKY EATERS

The best place to begin for a picky eater is with a slightly heavy fruit mixture that is quite sweet. Kids, as you know, tend to like things that are sweet. My friend Haynes calls this the beginner smoothie and I love that!

The typical American child's taste buds are constantly bathed in sugar, affecting their taste preferences. Once we begin giving their bodies more of the vitamins, minerals, and phytonutrients they need in order for their cells to work properly, their taste buds often begin to shift, and their palate often naturally expands.

Over time, decrease the fruit content while increasing the vegetable content. Literally, you can add in one, two, and three leaves of lettuce, bok choy, or microgreens at a time. If your child is particular about the color of the smoothie, put it in an opaque cup with an opaque straw so they cannot see the color!

If your child will not drink a smoothie at first, let's see if we can get her to eat something with protein and fat in the morning instead of simple carbs and sugar (a waffle with syrup or cereal and cow's milk). Since everyone, even picky eaters, seems to like bacon, I'd rather she eat organic bacon for breakfast and maybe eventually a small smoothie, instead of cereal and milk.

SMOOTHIE BLENDING TIPS

Fresh greens. Blend more smoothly than frozen greens, but just use whatever you have on hand. It's also best to mix greens with your liquid *first* and then add the rest of the ingredients.

If your child has a robust GI system, meaning they have at least one formed bowel movement per day and rarely complain of stomachaches or bloating, you may use raw spinach, kale, dandelion greens, or any other dark green leafy vegetable for your smoothies. If your child has constipation or loose stools, bloating, or regular abdominal pain, start with lettuce, microgreens, or bok choy. They will be easier to digest at first. Once the stool becomes daily and easy and the abdominal pain has resolved, then you can start rotating in those other darker leafy greens which are full of vitamin K and folate.

Chia seeds. Consider soaking them for ten to fifteen minutes in three to four tablespoons of water before adding them to your smoothie. This makes them gelatinous, and they will mix better this way.

Coconut oil. It's liquid at room temperature, and at cooler temperatures, it is solid. If you add coconut oil to frozen fruit, it will become quite hard. If I am using any frozen fruit in my smoothies, I usually blend everything first and then add the coconut oil. This keeps it smoother and it blends better with the other ingredients. Remember, a small amount goes a long way. I would keep it to half a teaspoon or less.

SWEETENERS

If your child still needs a sweeter smoothie when you begin this process, consider adding a touch of honey or maple syrup.

Flavor enhancers to consider using: ginger, fresh lemon or lime juice, vanilla, and cacao powder.

ABOUT THESE RECIPES

The recipes included here were a team effort by three wonderful friends and health coaches: Haynes Paschall of The Right Bite and the sister duo, Adri Warrick and Carolyn Hallett, of the Whole Tulip. Please check out their websites. These ladies are incredible, and they are huge advocates in our community to help families take back their health and their nutrition!

BEGINNER SMOOTHIE:
banana berry heaven

MAKES 2-3 SMOOTHIES

3 lettuce leaves or 2-inch piece bok choy or
1 tablespoon microgreens (fresh blends the best)

1 banana, peeled and sliced (fresh or frozen)

1 cup frozen berries
(strawberries or raspberries are a good start) or 1 peeled orange

1 cup water or 1 cup non-dairy milk
(e.g., organic coconut, rice, hemp, or almond)

Add the greens, banana, berries, and liquid of choice to a blender and blend until smooth. As your child gets used to this smoothie, enlist his or her help in preparing the intermediate smoothies that follow.

You may also increase the amount of "green" in this smoothie by adding 1 or 2 spinach leaves each time you make it. Letting your child be the one to add the leaves will encourage his or her interest in the smoothie becoming more and more "green."

INTERMEDIATE SMOOTHIE:
pina colada

MAKES 2-3 SMOOTHIES

2 cups lettuce, bok choy, or microgreens (fresh blends the best)

2 cups coconut milk

1 teaspoon chia seeds (soaked for 5 to 10 minutes or overnight)

1 cup pineapple chunks

1 cup frozen mango

2 bananas, peeled and sliced

1 tablespoon coconut oil

Add the greens, coconut milk, chia seeds, pineapple, frozen mango, bananas, and coconut oil to a blender and blend until smooth.

If the coconut oil doesn't blend smoothly, try mixing all of the other ingredients together first. Then add the coconut oil and blend into the mixture.

INTERMEDIATE SMOOTHIE:
cilantro-mango detox green

This recipe comes from Jen Hansard, website Simple Green Smoothies.

This smoothie is one of my favorites!

MAKES 2–3 SMOOTHIES

1½ cups spinach, fresh

½ cup cilantro, fresh

2 cups water

1½ cups frozen mango

1 cup pineapple chunks

1 tablespoon chia seeds (soaked for 5 to 10 minutes or overnight)

½ avocado, peeled and chopped

Add the spinach, cilantro, water, mango, pineapple, chia seeds, and avocado to a blender and blend until smooth.

jolly green smoothie

MAKES 2–3 SMOOTHIES

1 banana, peeled and sliced (frozen is preferable)

1 cup frozen raspberries

1 cup frozen strawberries

1 big handful of spinach, fresh

½ orange or 1 clementine, peeled and separated

1 tablespoon chia or flaxseeds

1 tablespoon maca (optional)

2 cups unsweetened vanilla almond milk

Add the banana, raspberries, strawberries, spinach, orange or clementine, chia/flaxseeds, maca, and almond milk to a blender and blend until smooth and a beautiful red color.

rockin' cacao smoothie

MAKES 1–2 SMOOTHIES

1 cup ice

1 banana, peeled and sliced

3 tablespoons raw cacao powder

3 dates (pitted)

1 tablespoon chia seeds

1 cup unsweetened coconut milk
(enough to cover the base of your smoothie)

Add the ice, banana, cacao powder, dates, chia seeds, and coconut milk to a blender and blend until smooth. Add more liquid or ice to achieve the desired consistency.

cashew milk

MAKES ABOUT 4 CUPS

ITEMS NEEDED

Cheesecloth (at least two pieces)
Strainer

1 cup raw cashews
4 cups filtered water, plus 2 cups for soaking
1 teaspoon vanilla extract
Pinch of sea salt

In a large glass bowl, soak the nuts in 2 cups of filtered water overnight.

Drain off the water in the morning and put the nuts in a blender with the remaining 4 cups of filtered water. Add the vanilla and salt. Blend for 3 minutes on high speed.

Cover the large strainer with two layers of cheesecloth and hold it over a large bowl that has a pouring spout.

Pour the contents of the blender through the strainer and catch the milk in the bowl. Wrap the cheesecloth around the pulp and squeeze out any excess water.

Pour the milk into a glass jar with a tight lid. Any unused milk can be stored in the refrigerator for 3 to 4 days.

Shake before using.

NOTE:
You may be able to find a recipe online to make something with the pulp. I once made delicious carrot cake with the pulp from juiced carrots!

breakfasts

baked eggs in a muffin tin

From Haynes Paschall of The Right Bite

Shhh . . . . The kids may think the sweet potato is cheese! For children who are still learning to love veggies, skip the onion and red pepper. The sweet potato and coconut milk give this recipe a pleasantly sweet flavor.

MAKES 6 SERVINGS

2 tablespoons coconut oil, divided

5 farm-fresh eggs

¼ cup unsweetened coconut milk

Salt and pepper to taste

½ cup sweet potato, peeled and grated

¼ cup onion, diced

¼ cup red bell pepper, diced

Preheat the oven to 350 degrees.

Grease 6 muffin tins with 1 tablespoon of coconut oil.

Whisk the eggs, coconut milk, and salt and pepper, and set aside.

Sauté the sweet potato, onion, and bell pepper in 1 tablespoon of coconut oil over medium heat, for 5 to 7 minutes or until soft.

Stir the sautéed veggies into the egg mixture. Pour evenly into the greased muffin tins. Each cup should be about ¾ full. Bake for 12 to 15 minutes, rotating the pan after 8 minutes, until the eggs are set in the center and a fork inserted into the middle of a muffin comes out clean.

Leftovers can be stored in the refrigerator and reheated as needed.

quinoa breakfast cereal

MAKES 4 SERVINGS

1 cup organic non-dairy milk

1 cup water

1 cup organic quinoa

1 tablespoon chia seeds

1 cup fresh or frozen blueberries

½ teaspoon ground cinnamon

Honey to taste

In a medium saucepan, combine the milk, water, and quinoa. Bring to a boil over high heat. Reduce the heat and cover. Simmer for 15 minutes or until most of the liquid is absorbed. Turn off the heat, stir in the chia seeds, and let stand covered for 5 minutes. Stir in the blueberries and cinnamon. Add honey to taste.

apple chia seed pudding

MAKES 2 SERVINGS

2 cups unsweetened non-dairy milk

½ teaspoon vanilla extract

⅔ cup chia seeds

2 tablespoons unsweetened coconut flakes

2 apples, cored and chopped

2 teaspoons cinnamon

WARM CHIA SEED PUDDING:

Place the milk and vanilla extract in a medium saucepan and warm over low heat for 2 to 3 minutes. The milk does not have to be boiling hot, just warm enough for your taste. Add the chia seeds to a cereal bowl. When the milk is warm, add the milk to your bowl of chia seeds. Stir continuously for about 2 minutes, while the chia seeds absorb the milk. Allow the mixture to sit for 2 to 3 minutes. Top with the coconut flakes, apple slices, and cinnamon.

ROOM-TEMPERATURE CHIA SEED PUDDING:

Add the milk to your bowl of chia seeds. Stir until the chia seeds have absorbed the milk (about 3 to 5 minutes). Top with the coconut flakes, apples, and cinnamon.

easy paleo pancakes

MAKES 1 SERVING

1 banana, peeled and mashed

2 farm-fresh eggs, whisked

Stir the banana and eggs together until well combined.

Fry the mixture in ghee or coconut oil.

You also can make a big batch of pancakes and freeze them.

scrambled eggs and smashed potatoes

MAKES 6 SERVINGS

4 white potatoes

Ghee

¼ to ½ cup warmed nut milk (optional)

6 fresh-farm eggs

1 red, sweet, and slightly hot habañero pepper, seeded and diced

2 handfuls of microgreens, chopped

1–2 tablespoons of water

Salt and pepper to taste

SMASHED POTATOES:

Wash and cut the potatoes into fourths, leaving the skin on.

Place them in a small pot of boiling water until they are soft (about 20 to 30 minutes).

Drain the water and smash the potatoes with a hand masher.

Add ghee (or butter) and salt to taste. If you don't want to use nut milk, you can add a little water to soften the smashed potatoes.

SCRAMBLED EGGS WITH PEPPERS AND MICROGREENS:
Heat a cast-iron skillet with a small amount of ghee (enough to cover the bottom of the skillet).

Scramble the eggs in a bowl, add the diced habañero peppers, chopped microgreens, a small amount of water (1 to 2 tablespoons), and salt and pepper. Pour the mixture into the skillet and cook until the eggs are firm.

Serve with a handful of fresh microgreens and hot tea.

> **NOTES:**
> *If you're casein free, consider using ghee instead of butter, because the butter may contain trace amounts of casein.*
>
> *If you feel like you need a piece of toast, try a warmed organic corn tortilla. I heat these directly over the open flame on my gas stove.*

magnesium muffins

This recipe comes from Andi Stowe, website Nourished Blessings

MAKES 8-12 MUFFINS

3 cups baked sweet potato or 2 15-ounce cans
of organic pumpkin pie filling

4 farm-fresh eggs, room temp;
5 farm-fresh eggs if using pumpkin pie filling

½ cup honey (amount can be decreased,
based on personal preference)

⅓ cup coconut oil, melted

½-pound bag raw pumpkin seeds (without shells)

1 teaspoon baking soda

¾ teaspoon ground cinnamon

½ teaspoon ground nutmeg

¼ teaspoon ground ginger

¼ teaspoon ground sea salt

Enjoy Life Gluten-Free Dairy-Free Mini Chocolate Chips (optional)

Preheat the oven to 350 degrees.

Bake the whole sweet potatoes until tender. Allow to cool completely, then peel and chop.

Blend the sweet potato or pumpkin pie filling, eggs, honey, and coconut oil in a high-powered blender until well combined.

Add the pumpkin seeds to the sweet potato/pumpkin mixture and blend until smooth.

In a small bowl, mix the baking soda, cinnamon, nutmeg, ginger, and sea salt, and slowly combine with the sweet potato/pumpkin mixture.

If you want to include the chocolate chips, chill the batter before folding the chips into the mixture.

Pour the mixture into a lined muffin pan and bake 20 to 30 minutes or until a toothpick inserted in the center of a muffin comes out clean.

NOTES:

If you use pumpkin pie filling instead of sweet potatoes, bake for 28 to 35 minutes.

Caution: Pumpkin seeds are high in magnesium and thus act as a laxative.

magnesium muffins—egg-free

This recipe comes from Andi Stowe, website Nourished Blessings

MAKES 8–12 MUFFINS

1 tablespoon ground psyllium husk

2 tablespoons water

3 cups baked sweet potato

4 psyllium husk "eggs"

½ cup honey (or much less, depending on taste)

⅓ cup coconut oil (melted)

½-pound bag raw pumpkin seeds (without shells)

1 teaspoon baking soda

¾ teaspoon ground cinnamon

½ teaspoon ground nutmeg

¼ teaspoon ground ginger

¼ teaspoon ground sea salt

Preheat the oven to 350 degrees.

To make the "eggs," mix the psyllium husk and water together, then set aside.

(recipe continues)

Bake the whole sweet potatoes until tender. Allow to cool until warm, then peel and chop.

Blend the "eggs," honey, coconut oil, and pumpkin seeds in a high-powered blender until well combined.

Add the warm sweet potato to the blender and mix until smooth.

In a medium bowl, mix the baking soda, cinnamon, nutmeg, ginger, and sea salt. Blend on low with the sweet potato mixture.

Pour the mixture into a lined muffin pan and bake for 20 to 30 minutes or until a toothpick inserted in the middle of a muffin comes out clean.

NOTE:

Caution: Pumpkin seeds are high in magnesium and psyllium husks act as a laxative.

five lunches or dinners

gluten-free chicken fingers

This recipe is from Leanne Ely, website Saving Dinner

MAKES 4 SERVINGS

2 farm-fresh eggs

½ cup coconut flour

1 teaspoon paprika

½ teaspoon garlic powder

½ teaspoon salt

¼ teaspoon pepper

¾ cup unsweetened shredded coconut

1 pound organic chicken tenderloins

Preheat the oven to 400 degrees.

Whisk the eggs in a medium bowl. In a second bowl mix the coconut flour, paprika, garlic powder, salt, and pepper. In a third bowl, place the shredded coconut.

Take one chicken tenderloin at a time and dip it into the eggs, then into the coconut flour mixture. Dip the tenderloin in the egg mixture again, and then in the shredded coconut.

Place the coated tenders on a baking pan lined with parchment paper or a wire rack that fits on a baking sheet. Bake for 20 minutes, flipping the tenders at the 10-minute mark. When done, the chicken tenders will be golden brown and completely cooked through.

potato soup

From Haynes Paschall of The Right Bite

MAKES 6-8 SERVINGS

This dairy-free soup gets its creaminess from cauliflower. Picky eaters will never know! This dish can be made on the stovetop or in a slow cooker.

8 cups organic chicken or vegetable broth

1 head cauliflower, washed and chopped

2-3 pounds Yukon gold potatoes, washed and chopped

2 garlic cloves, minced

1 onion, diced

1-2 teaspoons salt

Pepper to taste

Bring the broth to simmer in a large pot. Add the cauliflower, potatoes, garlic, onion, salt, and pepper and bring to a boil. Reduce the heat and simmer for 30 minutes or until the potato and cauliflower are tender and break apart easily. Let the soup cool for 10 minutes, then blend with an immersion blender or blend in small quantities in a regular countertop blender.

This soup can also be made in a slow cooker. Place all ingredients in the cooker and cook on low for 6 to 8 hours, then blend with immersion or countertop blender.

turkey chili

MAKES 4 SERVINGS

2 tablespoons extra virgin olive oil

½ cup white onion, diced

1 pound organic ground turkey

1 15-ounce can organic cannellini beans

1 16-ounce can or jar organic crushed tomatoes

½ cup of organic chicken broth

1 tablespoon chili powder

1 teaspoon red pepper flakes

1 tablespoon turmeric powder

Salt and pepper to taste

Heat the olive oil in a large pot over medium heat. Add the onions and sauté for 3 to 4 minutes. Add the ground turkey and cook all the way through. Add the cannellini beans, crushed tomatoes, and chicken broth, and combine well. Stir in the chili powder, red pepper flakes, turmeric, salt, and pepper. Cover with a lid and let simmer until ready to serve. Adjust seasoning and thickness as needed.

quinoa fried rice

MAKES 4 SERVINGS

4 cups cooked and chilled quinoa

3 tablespoons ghee

2 eggs, whisked

2 medium carrots, peeled and diced

1 small white onion, diced

½ cup frozen peas

3 garlic cloves, minced

Salt and pepper to taste

3–4 tablespoons gluten-free tamari, or more to taste

½ cup pineapple, diced

½ teaspoon toasted sesame oil

Prepare the quinoa as directed on the package. After it is fully cooked, allow it to cool and then chill in a refrigerator.

(recipe continues)

Heat ½ tablespoon of the ghee in a large skillet over medium-high heat until melted. Add the eggs and cook until scrambled, stirring occasionally. Remove the egg and transfer to a separate container.

Add an additional 1 tablespoon of ghee to the pan and heat until melted. Add the carrots, onion, peas, and garlic, and season with a generous pinch of salt and pepper. Sauté for about 5 minutes or until the onion and carrots are soft.

Increase heat to high, add in the remaining 1½ tablespoons of ghee, and stir until melted. Immediately add the cooked quinoa, tamari, and pineapple. Stir until combined. Continue stirring for an additional 3 minutes to fry the quinoa. Add the eggs and stir to combine.

Add the sesame oil, stir to combine, and remove from heat.

Serve warm.

kid-approved zucchini, squash, and snap pea stir fry

MAKES 4 SERVINGS

2 organic chicken breasts

1 zucchini, rinsed and sliced thin

1 squash, rinsed and sliced thin

1 cup snap peas

1 head broccoli, chopped

1 box rice noodles

2–3 tablespoons gluten-free tamari sauce
or Bragg's Liquid Aminos

Handful of basil leaves, chopped

Cut the chicken into bite-size pieces. Marinate for 1 hour or longer in your favorite gluten-free marinade.

While the chicken marinates, boil a pot of water for the rice noodles.

Heat the ghee in a sauté pan and add the zucchini, squash, snap peas, and broccoli, stirring frequently.

Heat ghee in another sauté pan and add the chicken. Cook the chicken 5 to 7 minutes, until cooked all the way through.

Add the rice noodles to the boiling water and prepare as directed on the package.

Add the cooked chicken and noodles to the veggie pan and toss with 2 to 3 tablespoons of the tamari or Bragg's Liquid Aminos. Add the chopped basil. Add additional tamari sauce if desired.

Serve hot.

five dinners and five side dishes

chicken vegetable soup and sweet potato fries

MAKES 2 SERVINGS

CHICKEN VEGETABLE SOUP

½ medium onion, chopped

2 large carrots, peeled and chopped

3 celery stalks, chopped

1 cup uncooked wild rice, rinsed and drained

1 bay leaf

½ teaspoon dried thyme or 1 tablespoon fresh thyme

Salt and black pepper, to taste

1 organic chicken breast

4 cups low-sodium organic chicken broth

In a slow cooker, combine the onion, carrots, celery, wild rice, bay leaf, thyme, salt, and pepper. Top with the chicken breast. Add the chicken broth.

Place the lid on the slow cooker and cook on low heat for 8 hours or on high heat about 4 hours.

Remove the chicken and shred it with two forks. Return it to the slow cooker and stir. Remove the bay leaf. Add salt and pepper to taste.

SWEET POTATO FRIES

1 large sweet potato, peeled

Olive oil

Salt to taste

Preheat the oven to 375 degrees.

Rinse and slice the sweet potato into thin slices like a French fry. Lightly coat with olive oil. Sprinkle with salt.

Cook 15 to 20 minutes or until the fries start to brown and are slightly crunchy.

turkey kale soup

MAKES 4 SERVINGS

1 tablespoon olive oil

4 celery stalks, thinly sliced

½ onion, chopped

3 large carrots, peeled and chopped

Salt and pepper to taste

1 pound organic ground turkey

1 tablespoon tomato paste

1 16-ounce can crushed tomatoes

1 16-ounce can cannellini beans, drained and rinsed (optional)

4 cups organic low-sodium chicken stock

1 teaspoon Italian seasoning

3 cups kale, stems removed and roughly chopped into ribbons

In a large, heavy-bottomed pot, heat the olive oil over medium heat. Add the celery, onion, and carrot, and a little salt and pepper, and sauté until the onions are translucent and the carrots and celery are soft.

Add the ground turkey and a little more salt and pepper to give the turkey some flavor. Stir often until the turkey is cooked through. You might need to move the vegetables to the sides of the pan and get some heat to it before working it into the vegetables.

(recipe continues)

After the turkey is cooked through, stir in the tomato paste and let cook for a few minutes, stirring frequently so the tomato paste doesn't burn. Add the crushed tomatoes, cannellini beans, and chicken stock. Bring to a boil and let simmer for 20 to 25 minutes.

Before you are ready to serve, stir in the kale and let it wilt. Season with salt and pepper to taste and serve.

lentil tacos

From Haynes Paschall of The Right Bite

MAKES 8-10 SERVINGS

1½ cups dried lentils

2 cups vegetable broth (or more as needed)

2 tablespoons coconut oil

½ onion, chopped

2 carrots, diced

3 garlic cloves, minced

1 teaspoon ground cumin

1 teaspoon cayenne pepper

1 teaspoon chili powder

Salsa (optional)

Guacamole (optional)

Combine lentils and vegetable broth in a medium pot and bring to a boil. Reduce the heat to low and cover. Simmer 30 to 40 minutes, stirring occasionally, until desired consistency is reached. Add more broth as needed, so the lentils do not stick to the pan and burn.

In a separate pot, sauté the onion and carrots in coconut oil over medium heat until soft, about 10 minutes. Add the garlic, cumin, cayenne pepper, and chili powder and cook another 3 minutes.

When the lentils have reached the desired consistency, combine them with the onion/carrot/spice mixture.

Serve with crunchy organic corn taco shells, with soft corn shells, or over a salad. Top with salsa and guacamole if desired.

teriyaki salmon

MAKES 4 SERVINGS

¼ cup gluten-free tamari
1 teaspoon sesame oil
1 orange, juiced (about ¼ cup)
1 tablespoon honey
1 tablespoon grated ginger
4 wild-caught salmon filets

First, make the teriyaki sauce by whisking together the tamari, sesame oil, orange juice, honey, and grated ginger in a bowl. Place the salmon in an oven-safe casserole dish, skin-side down. Baste the salmon with some of the teriyaki sauce and place the dish on the top oven rack. Turn the oven on and set it to a low broil (high broil will cook it too quickly and make it tough). Let the salmon cook for about 5 minutes, then baste the salmon with more teriyaki sauce. Keep basting the salmon every few minutes until cooked to desired doneness.

turmeric rice

MAKES 4 SERVINGS

1 cup rice

2¼ cups water

1½ tablespoons coconut oil or ghee

1 tablespoon turmeric powder, more to taste

¼ teaspoon ground black pepper

Sea salt to taste (Himalayan sea salt is preferable)

4 to 6 cardamom seeds (whole, dried)

A handful of raisins (optional)

½ cup broccoli chopped into small pieces—
add into rice with about 5 minutes left of cooking

¾ to 1 cup of spinach, chopped—
stir in after the rice has cooked and while it is still hot

1 cup of organic cooked chicken chopped and mixed in (optional)

This can be made in a rice cooker or on the stove just as you would cook rice. Follow the instructions on the package for the rice. You may need to add a bit more water than what the rice package indicates.

NOTES:

I often use basmati or jasmine rice, but brown or black rice has a lower glycemic index.

Although the black pepper facilitates absorption of the turmeric, those with Crohn's disease or ulcerative colitis should leave out the black pepper, because this allows the turmeric to remain within the GI system and carry out its anti-inflammatory properties where it's needed most—in the gut.

baked kale

MAKES 4 SERVINGS

One bundle of fresh, organic kale
Olive oil for drizzle
Salt to taste

Preheat the oven to 250 degrees.

Wash and cut the kale. You can use kitchen scissors to cut the kale into about 2-inch pieces, cutting off the thick stems.

Spread the kale on a baking sheet.

Sprinkle olive oil over the leaves

Bake for about 15 to 20 minutes. If the pieces are not as crisp as you like, turn the oven off, close the door for 5 more minutes, and then check them.

Salt to taste and enjoy.

baked beets

MAKES 4 SERVINGS

2 beets, washed and sliced
Ghee, melted for drizzle

Preheat the oven to 375 degrees.

Spread the beets out on a baking sheet.

Sprinkle the beets with the ghee. Since beets are baked at a higher temperature, and the smoking point of ghee is higher than olive oil, ghee is used for a little flavor and fat.

(recipe continues)

Bake for 20 to 30 minutes.

Salt to taste and enjoy!

NOTES:

I usually don't peel the beets if they're organic. I cut the beet in half and then make thick slices from each half.

Be aware that what comes out of your body over the next several days may look very purplish!

baked broccoli and cauliflower

MAKES 4 SERVINGS WITH LEFTOVERS

1 head organic fresh broccoli
1 head organic fresh cauliflower
1 tablespoon ghee, softened
Pinch of sea salt (Himalayan preferable)
Fresh ground black pepper
Turmeric powder to taste (optional)

Preheat the oven to 475 degrees.

Wash and chop the broccoli and cauliflower into small pieces that are easy for children's small fingers to pick up. Toss the pieces in a bowl with the softened ghee.

Spread the broccoli and cauliflower in one layer on a baking sheet.

Sprinkle with sea salt and ground black pepper. Bake for 10 to 15 minutes.

NOTES:

The ghee provides a small amount of saturated fat, which will help your child absorb the nutrients from the veggies.

If you're feeling adventurous, you could add a small amount of turmeric to the ghee to add a powerful anti-inflammatory spice and a great taste!

crispy chickpeas

MAKES 6 SERVINGS

4 15-ounce cans organic chickpeas
4 tablespoons extra virgin olive oil
Sea salt to taste

Preheat the oven to 400 degrees.

Rinse the beans, drain, and pat dry. Place them on a cookie sheet in one even layer. Drizzle with olive oil and toss until coated. You also can put the chickpeas in a bowl and toss with olive oil before you place them in the pan, but if you want to save a dish, coat them with olive oil on the pan.

Sprinkle with sea salt (add more later if desired).

Bake for 30 minutes or until desired crispiness is reached. Shake the pan a few times as the chickpeas cook. You may also want to add more olive oil during the baking process.

NOTES:

Make sure the chickpea can is BPA free, or prepare your own dry beans.

Coconut oil can be substituted for olive oil but does have a slightly different flavor.

Crispy chickpeas make a delicious salad or soup topper! You can also experiment with adding additional spices like turmeric, chili powder, or paprika. And don't forget to save leftovers! Kids love these in their lunchboxes.

desserts

almond meal cookies

MAKES 8–12 COOKIES

1 cup almond meal

1 teaspoon ground cardamom

1 teaspoon ground cinnamon

2 tablespoons water

¼ cup maple syrup

Preheat the oven to 350 degrees.

Combine the almond meal, cardamom, cinnamon, water, and maple syrup and form the mixture into balls. Place on a baking sheet. Bake for 15 minutes or to desired crispiness.

no-bake energy balls

MAKES 18–24

1 cup gluten-free oats

1 cup unsweetened shredded coconut

½ cup dark chocolate chips (try to get 60% or higher cacao)

½ cup peanut butter, sunflower seed butter, or another nut butter
(organic and no added sugars, oils, or corn syrup)

½ cup ground flaxseed

⅓ cup raw honey (try to use local and raw)

1 teaspoon vanilla

Mix the oats, coconut, chocolate chips, peanut butter, flaxseed, honey, and vanilla together. Chill the mixture for an hour, and then form into balls.

Energy balls can be stored in the refrigerator for up to one week.

chocolate sunflower butter protein balls

A fabulous perk of these protein balls is that they're allergy-friendly, so you can send them to schools that don't allow nuts.

MAKES 12–18

6 tablespoons sunflower seed butter

4 tablespoons raw cacao

2 tablespoons coconut oil

1 tablespoon ground flaxseed, chia seeds, or almond meal

2 tablespoons hemp seeds

1 tablespoon honey

Pinch of sea salt

1 cup unsweetened shredded coconut

Water (as needed)

Combine the sunflower seed butter, cacao, coconut oil, ground flaxseed/chia seeds/almond meal, hemp seeds, honey, sea salt, and coconut in a large bowl.

Stir and add water ¼ teaspoon at a time, until you get the desired consistency for the protein balls. The mixture should be thick and easily roll into a ball. If the mixture is too thin, refrigerate it for 30 minutes to 1 hour and let it harden.

Roll the dough into little balls and place them on a cookie sheet or wax paper.

(recipe continues)

Place the coconut in a bowl and roll each ball in the coconut. Feel free to dust the balls with more cacao for an extra boost of antioxidants.

You can eat the balls right away or freeze them for 10–15 minutes.

strawberry, banana, and peanut butter popsicles

MAKES ABOUT 12 POPSICLES

1½ cups frozen organic strawberries

1 banana, peeled and sliced

3 tablespoons peanut butter or other nut butter

1 tablespoon chia seeds

1½ to 2 cups unsweetened vanilla almond milk or unsweetened coconut milk

Add the strawberries, banana, peanut butter, chia seeds, and almond/coconut milk to a blender. Blend until smooth and creamy. Pour into popsicle molds and freeze overnight.

chocolate banana pudding

MAKES 1 SERVING

4 tablespoons chia seeds

1 cup non-dairy milk (hemp, coconut, or almond)

1 small banana, peeled and mashed

1 heaping teaspoon raw cacao

Honey to taste

Hemp seeds for garnish (optional)

Shredded coconut for garnish (optional)

For best results, combine the chia seeds, non-dairy milk, banana, and cacao the night before and let the mixture set in the refrigerator. The next morning, you can eat the pudding cold.

If you prefer the pudding warm, simply heat the non-dairy milk in the morning make sure the milk is warm, not boiling. While the milk warms up, mix the chia seeds, banana, and cacao in a bowl. Add the milk to the bowl and stir well.

For either the cold or warm option, you can add honey, hemp seeds, and shredded coconut.

DR. KILBANE'S APPROVED PACKAGED FOODS

Food manufacturers frequently change product ingredients. Please always double check what you are buying. Not all of these products are organic. Keep non-organic products to a minimum.

Condiments
Primal Kitchen condiments
Tessemae's dressings
New Primal condiments
Kite Hill
Hope Cashew and Almond Dip
Hope Hummus
Bulletproof Products (Brain Octane Oil)

Snacks
Siete grain-free chips
The New Primal Jerky
Kite Hill almond cream cheese and Greek yogurt
Simple Mills Crackers
Primal Kitchen Bars
Larabar
Forager Unsweetened Cashew Yogurt
So Delicious Unsweetened Coconut Yogurt
Purely Elizabeth Grain-Free Granola
Nativas Organics Power Snacks
Lesser Evil Paleo Puffs
Mavuno Harvest Organic Dried Fruit
Chomp's Jerky
Hu Grain-Free Crackers

Sides and Mains
Jovial Organic Pasta
Banza Pasta
Birch Benders Gluten Free pancake and waffle mix

Applegate Natural & Organic Meats
Daily Harvest Ready-To-Blend Smoothies
Cappello's grain-free pizza crust and pasta
Sprouted for Life Gluten-Free Bread

Sweets
Simple Mills Gluten Free baking mixes
Enjoy Life Dark Chocolate Chips
Eating Evolved Chocolate
Hu Kitchen Chocolate
NadaMoo! Coconut milk ice cream

Drinks
Pay attention to the sugar content of flavored milks
   (chocolate or vanilla)
Califia Farms organic non-dairy milks
Elmhurst non-dairy milks
MALK organic non-dairy milks
New Barn organic non-dairy milks
Oatly organic non-dairy milks
Simple Truth organic non-dairy milks
Three Trees organic non-dairy milks
Thrive Market organic non-dairy milks

Electrolyte Drink
Ultima Replenisher

(List created in collaboration with my amazing hair stylist, Brooke Ridberg, mother of three.)

appendix

healthy kids happy moms - SYMPTOM TRACKER*

We will use this tracking tool to assess your child's
symptoms and progress throughout the program.

The most important number to follow is the TOTAL at the bottom. As your child's
symptoms begin to improve, this number should decrease. If you want to share your
child's progress on the closed Facebook group - Dr. Kilbane's Healthy Kids Happy Moms
Book Club (along with before and after pictures of your child) for support and
encouragement, please do! We can do this together!

None = 0	Mild = 1 or 2	Moderate = 2 or 3	Severe = 4 or 5

Abnormal bowel movements   _____

Abdominal pain   _____

Headaches   _____

Poor sleep quality   _____

Mouth breathing or snoring   _____

Dark circles under the eyes   _____

Bumps on cheeks, arms, thighs   _____

Eczema   _____

Allergies   _____

Asthma   _____

Recurrent ear infections   _____

Recurrent sinus infections   _____

Meltdowns or mood swings   _____

TOTAL   _____   DATE _____

Stopped or decreased any prescription or over-the-counter meds?

☐ No
☐ Yes

If yes, What medication? _____

New dose? _____

Consistency with nutrition and supplements this week?

☐ 100% We were total rock stars! 😎

☐ 75% We were quite good! ✋

☐ 25% We had some other priorities but are still doing better than before the cleanse! 📋

☐ 0% We had a full life outside of supplements and green smoothies. 😜

* This is a tool to be used solely for tracking symptoms over time. It has not been scientifically validated.

GUT HEALTH
Antibiotics and Probiotics

Antibiotics kill the bacteria in our ears, lungs, or sinuses that cause acute infection and are highly necessary at times. However, they also can impact the beneficial bacteria in the gut. If your child needs to take an antibiotic, it's important to follow your doctor's guidance and take the antibiotic. You may also consider adding in a probiotic (and/or fermented and prebiotic foods). See list of foods that contain prebiotics and probiotics and are high in fiber.

A five- to ten-day course of antibiotics can impact the gut bacteria anywhere from six months to a year.[1,2] I recommend my patients take a probiotic while they are taking an antibiotic to support the gut environment. Probiotics can also help prevent antibiotic-associated diarrhea and the yeast-driven diaper rash or vaginal irritation that can sometimes accompany a round of antibiotics.[3] We need more research in this area, but this is how I advise my patients currently.

HOW TO TAKE A PROBIOTIC
WHEN TAKING AN ANTIBIOTIC

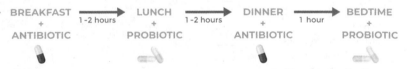

BREAKFAST + ANTIBIOTIC		LUNCH + PROBIOTIC		DINNER + ANTIBIOTIC		BEDTIME + PROBIOTIC
	1-2 hours		1-2 hours		1 hour	

Take the probiotic 1 to 2 hours before or after taking the antibiotic.
Please modify if the antibiotic has to be taken 3 or 4 times a day.
Continue the probiotic for at least two months after you stop the antibiotic.

 Research is rapidly changing

 Discuss with your doctor

FOODS THAT SUPPORT THE HEALTH AND DIVERSITY OF THE MICROBIOME

Foods That Contain Probiotics

Fermented foods, not pickled foods. Fermented foods contain beneficial bacteria and yeast. Fermentation takes time whereas pickling uses vinegar.

Pickles (be sure they don't contain high-fructose corn syrup or vinegar)

Sauerkraut

Kimchi

Kombucha

Tempeh, natto, and miso (soy based)

Yogurt (non-dairy for those who are sensitive or allergic to dairy)

Often with my patients, the family is just beginning to make major shifts in diet and lifestyle. If the probiotic- and prebiotic-rich foods aren't commonplace, we use a probiotic supplement while we begin incorporating some of these foods into the diet.

 Proceed with caution

Fermented foods and some probiotics can increase histamine levels in the body for some people, making symptoms (such as bloating, gas, loose stools, and/or eczema) worse or even creating new symptoms.

Foods containing prebiotics
(food for the beneficial gut bacteria)

Bananas

Onion

Garlic

Chicory root

Dandelion greens

Jerusalem artichokes

Leeks

Asparagus

Apples

Jicama root

Chia seed

Flaxseed

Hemp seed

Vegetables, especially homegrown in the soil or purchased from a farmer (the soil is teeming with microorganisms that support our gut health)

Activities that support the microbiome

Playing outside in the dirt

Gardening

Being around animals

Spending time on a farm

Walking outside in the woods

MINI CLEANSE

Sugar 4 grams = 1 tsp

To figure out how many teaspoons of sugar are in a particular food, look at the number of grams of sugar and divide that by 4 (24 grams of sugar / 4 = 6 teaspoons).

American Heart Association (AHA) Guidelines on Daily Sugar Intake[4]

AGE	2 TO 18 YEARS	ADULT WOMEN	ADULT MEN
Recommended Upper Limit of Teaspoons daily	4 to 6 (16 to 24 grams)	6	9
The Actual Average Daily Intake in Teaspoons[5]	12 to 34 (teenagers have the highest intake)		

Sugar Content of Common Beverages Kids Drink

TWELVE-OUNCE BEVERAGE	SUGAR (GRAMS)	NUMBER OF TEASPOONS
Can of soda	39	9¾
Orange juice	28	7
Cow's milk	19½	4¾
Vitamin Water (ten ounces)	16	4
Soy milk	14	3½
Almond milk, unsweetened	< 1	< 1

Notice how much sugar your child has ingested after eating a bowl of cereal with milk and a glass of orange juice in the morning.

Oils to Avoid and Their Healthy Replacements

OILS TO AVOID	OILS BEST FOR LOW OR NO HEAT COOKING	OILS SAFE FOR HIGH HEAT COOKING
Canola oil Grapeseed oil Rice bran oil "Vegetable" oil Safflower oil Soybean oil Corn oil Cottonseed oil	Olive oil Coconut oil Butter	Avocado oil Ghee (clarified butter)

High-Fiber Foods

VEGETABLES	FRUITS	SEEDS	NUTS	LEGUMES
Asparagus Broccoli Brussels sprouts Cauliflower Eggplant Onion Sweet potato Sugar beets Turnips	Apples Avocado Berries Grapefruit Oranges Pears Prunes	Chia Flaxseed Hemp Psyllium seed husk	Almonds (soaking before eating makes them easier to digest)	Beans Lentils Peas

Daily Fruit and Vegetable Recommendations

AGE	FRUIT CUPS PER DAY	VEGETABLES CUPS PER DAY
2 to 3 years	1	1
4 to 8 years	1 to 1½	1½
9 to 13 years (male)	1½	2½
9 to 13 years (female)	1½	2
14 to 18 years (male)	2	3
14 to 18 years (female)	1½	2½

Source: https://www.myplate.gov/eat-healthy/fruitshttps://www.myplate.gov/eat-healthy/fruits

Some helpful comparisons

2 medium carrots = 1 cup
3 medium stalks of celery = 1 cup
1 medium cucumber = 1½ cups
1 medium pepper chopped = ½ cup
1 small apple (tennis ball size) = 1 cup

2020 SHOPPER'S GUIDE TO PESTICIDES IN PRODUCE
Environmental Working Group (EWG.org)

By following this shoppers' guide for organic foods, you can reduce
your family's exposure to toxic chemicals by 92%.

EWG's 2020 Dirty 12™

1. Strawberries	7. Peaches
2. Spinach	8. Cherries
3. Kale	9. Pears
4. Nectarines	10. Tomatoes
5. Apples	11. Celery
6. Grapes	12. Potatoes

EWG's 2020 Clean 15™

1. Avocados	6. Sweet Peas (Frozen)	11. Broccoli
2. Sweet Corn	7. Eggplant	12. Mushrooms
3. Pineapple	8. Asparagus	13. Cabbage
4. Onions	9. Cauliflower	14. Honeydew Melon
5. Papaya	10. Cantaloupe	15. Kiwi

Removing Dairy/Gluten

Dietary Reference Intakes for Calcium
from the Institute of Medicine
Calcium expressed in milligrams per unit specified

0 to 6 months 200 mg/day	19 to 50 years 1,000 mg/day
6 to 12 months 260 mg/day	51 to 70 years (F) 1,200 mg/day
1 to 3 years 700 mg/day	51 to 70 years (M) 1,000 mg/day
4 to 8 years 1,000 mg/day	71+ years 1,200 mg/day
9 to 18 years 1,300 mg/day	

Calcium Content of Various Foods
Calcium expressed in milligrams per unit specified

Non-dairy Milks (Calcium per 1 Cup)

Many of these milks are fortified with calcium in the manufacturing process and
may vary from product to product. If you make them at home, please be aware that
the calcium content may be lower.

Oat	350	Quinoa	300
Hemp	300	Rice	290

Tree Nut Milks

Almond	480	Cashew	47
Coconut	460	Walnut	24

(coconut is actually a fruit, but the FDA labels it as a tree nut)

Legume Milk

Legumes can irritate the lining of the GI tract for some kids. These may not be good options for kids with significant GI issues or eczema.

Pea	440	Soy	300

Vegetables (calcium per 1 cup cooked unless otherwise specified)

Collard greens	265	Okra (raw)	80
Turnip greens	200	Broccoli microgreens (raw)	60 to 100
Mustard greens	165	Broccoli	60
Bok choy	160	Brussels sprouts	55
Beet greens	160	Acorn squash (raw)	45
Turnip greens	105	Watercress	40
Swiss chard	100	Carrots (raw)	40
Rhubarb	100	Asparagus	30
Broccoli rabe	100	Cauliflower (raw)	25
Kale	95	Red bell pepper (raw)	10
Winter squash	90	Spinach	250
Sweet potato	90	(Only a small percentage of the calcium in spinach is absorbed.)	
Butternut squash	85		

Fruit

Olives (1 cup)	100 to 190	Avocado (1 cup pureed)	30
Orange Juice (calcium-fortified)	290	Kiwi (1 large)	30
		Fig (1 large)	30
Orange (1 large)	75	Strawberries	25
Blackberries	40	Prunes (5)	20
Raspberries	30	Blueberries	10

Legumes (calcium per 1 cup canned)

Tofu	870	Hummus	90
Black-eyed peas	370	Snap peas (raw)	80
Mung beans	270	Green beans (cooked)	55
Kidney beans	260	Lentils	40
Soybeans	200	Peas (1 cup cooked)	40
White beans	190	Peanuts (¼ cup)	35
Chickpeas	210	Peanut butter (2 tablespoons)	15
Black beans	100		
Edamame	100		

Tree nuts (calcium per ¼ cup)

Almonds	95	Cashews	20
Pistachio	50	Walnuts	20

Seeds (calcium per 1 tablespoon)

Sesame	90	Flax	25
Tahini	65	Hemp	15
Chia	60		

Sweetener

Blackstrap molasses (1 tablespoon)   145

Plants/herbs

Stinging nettle (1 cup cooked)	450	Artichoke (1 large)	70
		Parsley (1 cup)	80

Gluten-free grains/flours (calcium per 1 cup)

Be sure the packaging says gluten-free.

Some grains can bother individuals with celiac disease or a gluten sensitivity. Be sure to pay attention to any GI upset, skin rash, or irritability if you decide to use any of these flours.

Teff	120	Quinoa	30
Amaranth	115	Sorghum	30
Steel cut oats	50	White rice	15
Buckwheat	30		

Animal products

Fish (canned with bones, calcium per 1 ounce)

Sardines	110	Salmon	80

Cooked animal products (calcium per 3 ounces)

Oysters	100	Beef	15
Shrimp	70	Pork	15
Herring	65	Lamb	15
Mackerel	65	Salmon	10
Mussels	30	Chicken	15
Egg (1 large)	25	Bone broth (1 cup)	10 to 70

Animal milks (calcium per 1 cup)

Goat's milk	330 (contains A2 beta-casein and very low amounts of A1 beta-casein)
Sheep's milk	475 (contains A2 beta-casein and almost no A1 beta-casein)

Cow's Milk Foods—Calcium Content for Comparison

Milk (1 cup)	300 (contains A1 beta-casein—can cause GI distress)[6]
Greek yogurt (3/4 cup)	190
Cheese (1 ounce)	200

SUPPLEMENT DOSING GUIDE

Please refer to my website sheilakilbane.com for an up-to-date list of the supplements I recommend, including dosing by age.

When possible, dosing is based upon the RDA or the AI. The RDA (recommended dietary allowance) is based upon scientific evidence and defined as the average daily dietary nutrient intake level sufficient to meet the needs of 98 percent of healthy individuals. AI (adequate intake) is established when evidence is insufficient to develop the RDA and it is set at a level assumed to ensure nutritional adequacy. You'll notice the omega-3 fat dosing is based upon the AI.

Problotic

Probiotics should *not* be given to anyone who is immunocompromised or who has venous access with a central line (an access port for those getting chemotherapy or long-term antibiotic infusions).

HKHM Plantadophilus

AGE	START OF BREAKFAST	START OF DINNER
Infants	Only under the guidance of a doctor	
1 year +	1 capsule	I capsule

You can open up the capsule and mix it with soft food, and it tastes surprisingly good!

For a list of foods that contain prebiotics and probiotics, see the Gut Health section of the Appendix.

Digestive Enzymes

Pick one form which will work best for your child: powder, chewable, or capsule.

HKHM Digest Powder (contains flax)

AGE	START OF BREAKFAST	START OF DINNER
Infants	Only under the guidance of a doctor	
1 to 2 years	half a scoop	half a scoop
3 years +	1 scoop	1 scoop

Take at the **start of breakfast and dinner along with the probiotic.**
May mix in soft food or liquid.

HKHM Kids Digest Chewable (contains flax)

AGE	START OF BREAKFAST	START OF DINNER
2 to 3 years	1 chewable	1 chewable
4 years +	2 chewable	2 chewable

HKHM Digest capsules

AGE	START OF BREAKFAST	START OF DINNER
3 to 5 years	½ capsule	½ capsule
6 years +	1 capsule	1 capsule

Enzyme That Helps Break Down Gluten

Dipeptidyl Peptidase IV (DPP-IV) enzyme: For those with celiac disease or a gluten sensitivity who are off gluten but continue to have symptoms.

HKHM CARBO-G

AGE	START OF BREAKFAST	START OF DINNER
3 to 5 years	½ capsule	½ capsule
6 years +	1 capsule	1 capsule

NATURAL WAYS TO IMPROVE DIGESTION

Do more of the activities that support digestion and fewer of the ones that compromise our digestion:

Be in a relaxed state when you are getting ready to eat.
Chew your food thoroughly.
Eat mindfully and slowly.
Eat with people you love.
Enhance your toolbox of ways to handle stress.
Eat foods that support the microbiome.
Cut out the processed, packaged, high-sugar foods.
Be sure you are having at least 1 daily, easy, formed bowel
   movement.

Omega-3 fats

The Current Recommended Adequate Intakes (AI) of Omega-3s for Kids

AGE	DOSE
0 to 12 months	500
1 to 3 years	700
4 to 8 years	900
9 to 13 years (male)	1,200
9 to 13 years (female)	1,000
14 to 10 years (male)	1,600
14 to 18 years (female)	1,100

Refer to my website sheilakilbane.com/book
for up-to-date and specific supplement suggestions

Omega-3 Foods

Coldwater fish: salmon, mackerel, herring, trout, char, sockeye, sardines

Flaxseeds, flax oil

Chia seeds

Hemp seeds

Walnuts

Almonds

(specify the meats)

Berries: blackberries, blueberries, strawberries

Brussels sprouts and other green leafy vegetables

Eggs (free range)

Vitamin D

Remember: Vitamin D is a fat-soluble vitamin which means you can overdose on it. Please follow the recommended guidelines unless advised by your doctor.

**Vitamin D Recommendations of
The American Academy of Pediatrics (AAP)
and The Institute of Medicine[7]**

AGE	DOSAGE
0 to 1 year	400 IUs/day
2 to 70 years	600 IUs/day
71 years +	800 IUs/day

Breastfeeding infants should be supplemented daily. Formula-fed babies who are not drinking one quart (thirty-two ounces) daily should be supplemented. Thirty-two ounces of formula contains 400 IU vitamin D.

Adequate vitamin D is extremely important for a developing baby. Studies show that less than 30 percent of US infants are getting adequate amounts, and breastfed babies were more likely to fall short of the guidelines than formula-fed babies.[8]

I typically give kids two years and older 1,000 IUs/day, but I also follow their levels via bloodwork. I try to keep my patient's levels between 40 and 60 ng/mL (100 to 150 nmol/L). This should only be done in conjunction with your child's doctor.

Refer to my website sheilakilbane.com/book
for up-to-date and specific supplement suggestions

How Do We Get Vitamin D Naturally?

We synthesize vitamin D through the absorption of sunlight from our skin. The amount of vitamin D we synthesize from the sun varies greatly and depends upon age, where you are in the world, the time of year, and skin pigmentation. Darker skin requires longer sun exposure. The time needed can range from ten minutes for a fair-skinned individual to sixty minutes for more pigmented skin. Sunscreen prevents the skin from synthesizing vitamin D.

A small number of foods contain vitamin D naturally.

Foods that Naturally Contain Vitamin D

	VITAMIN D[3] IU PER OUNCE
Blue fish	280
Cod	104
Grey sole	56
Salmon, Farm	240
Salmon, Wild	988
Trout, Farm	388
Ahi Tuna—Yellowfin	404

Vitamin D content varies from fish to fish and depending upon its source (farm raised have lower amounts than wild caught).

Foods Fortified with Vitamin D
(which means it doesn't occur naturally in that food)

Pasteurized milk, 100 IUs per 8 ounces

Orange juice, 100 IUs per 8 ounces

You'd have to drink more than 32 ounces daily of juice or milk to provide your body with the recommended amount of 600 IUs. I don't recommend anyone drink that much milk or juice in one day!

Whole-Food Supplement Options or Multivitamin Mineral Options (Pick One)

Multivitamin mineral supplements can be made from whole foods or synthetic based, meaning many of the ingredients are manufactured in a lab. My preference is for kids to supplement with products directly derived from food whenever possible.

Whole-Food Supplement Options
- Hiya Kids Daily Multivitamin
- Greens First Kids
- Garden of Life mykind Organics Kids Multi Gummies
- Vitamin Code Kids Chewable Whole Food Multivitamin
- JuicePLUS

or

Multivitamin Mineral Options
- Seeking Health Multivitamin Mineral
- Dr. Mercola Chewable Multivitamin for kids
- Smarty Pants Kids Complete

Refer to my website sheilakilbane.com/book for up-to-date and specific supplement suggestions

Magnesium

Magnesium RDA

AGE	MILLIGRAMS (MG) PER DAY
7 to 12 months	75
1 to 3 years	80
4 to 8 years	130
9 to 13 years	240
14 to 18 years (male)	410
14 to 18 years (female)	360
19 to 30 years (male)	400
19 to 30 years (female)	320
30 years + (male)	420
30 years + (female)	320

Your child may need a higher dose than what is listed if they have constipation or asthma. Magnesium supplements (in the right form) are safe and well-tolerated. You can dose magnesium to tolerance, which means if the stools become loose, decrease to a lower dose. You may titrate up or down for one soft stool per day.

 Refer to my website sheilakilbane.com/book for up-to-date and specific supplement suggestions

Foods High in Magnesium
- Green leafy vegetables (spinach)
- Nuts
- Seeds (pumpkin, chia, and flaxseed)

Sodas are high in phosphate which binds to magnesium, rendering it ineffective.

Many children (and adults) don't eat these foods on a daily basis, so magnesium supplementation can be extremely helpful. Many of the kids in my practice are on a magnesium supplement.

Zinc RDA

AGE	DOSE
0 to 6 months	2 mg
7 to 12 months	3 mg
1 to 2 years	3 mg
4 to 8 years	5 mg
9 to 13 years	8 mg
14 to 18 years (male)	11 mg
14 to 18 years (female)	9 mg
19 years + (male)	11 mg
19 years + (female)	8 mg

Do not give zinc longer than two months unless you are doing it in conjunction with your child's doctor.

 Refer to my website sheilakilbane.com/book for up-to-date and specific supplement suggestions

Foods High in Zinc

Oysters   Pumpkin seeds
Beef   Cashews
Crab   Almonds
Pork   Chickpeas
Chicken   Oats

acknowledgments

MY FIRST AND BIGGEST thank you is to my parents. Through their example, my four siblings and I learned how to live a life of service. I am forever grateful for their love and unconditional support in every way, shape, and form. They made me feel like I could do anything. They attended every single basketball game and track meet I ever participated in. They have been the constant presence of stability in my life. They even unpacked and organized my entire medical school apartment! They gave me business advice when I asked for it and a place to retreat when I needed a rest. Any success I've had in business and in life has been built on the foundation they created. I owe my ability to follow my gut to them. Best of all, they are quick-witted, fun, and know how to really enjoy life.

I have massive gratitude for the most supportive siblings, Karen, Tommy, Susan, and Michael, and my two in-laws, Pat and Lauren. They make me laugh, keep me humble, continue to call me by my childhood nicknames, and best of all, they have been my biggest cheerleaders from the get-go—thank you! This gratitude extends equally to each of their children, my dear nieces and nephews: Sean, Momo, Kathleen, Keara, Holden, Aidan, Liam, and Conor. This crew is amazing, and I have a really cool and unique bond with each of them. They are a big part of the fabric of my life, and I love them each to the moon and back!

My nephew Liam, my sister Susan, and my mother get a special shout-out for their editing prowess. I originally wrote this book in 2016 and, when I decided to revise it, I was on vacation with the entire clan. In the evenings, after everyone had gone to sleep, Liam, Susan, and my mother would sit with me at the long, wooden kitchen table in our cottage. They listened as I read aloud, offering me great suggestions, insights, and edits. Many Zoom calls later, we made it through the entire book.

Deb Allen is the integrative pharmacist who works with me in my private practice. This book took on a level of excellence that would not have been possible without her input, care, and brilliance.

My "extended family" here in Charlotte—the Schmelzers, Audinos, Mitras, Regans, Faircloths, Evans, Daniels, and Bumgarner-Phadkes—have listened to me yammer on about food and children's health for years. I couldn't be more grateful for all the belly laughs at the expense of two food categories, dairy and gluten. And an extra-special mention goes to John Evans for his gracious and copious editing. The man can find the most mundane grammar errors ever.

My dear friend Kristen Oliver taught me powerful tools to shift the way I experienced life. These concepts have allowed me to create things I never dreamed possible, including this book.

My incredible writing coach, Tamela Rich, provided the encouragement I needed to begin this journey. The mastermind group she led with four amazing women—Cathy, Lynne, Lou, and Suzanne—honed my writing skills. Tamela stepped in when I thought the book was almost finished but was twice as long as it needed to be. She spent hours in person and on Zoom, doing powerful developmental editing with me and helping make the book what it is today. Her patience, grace, and brilliance carried me across the finish line.

My rock star agents, Steve and Jan, believed in my work and my mission, and led me to the dream team at Harper Horizon: Andrea, Amanda, John, Leigh, and Jeff. Andrea, my publisher with Horizon, has been supportive beyond what I ever could have imagined. She clearly cares about the health of our children and has done everything in her power to set this book up to help as many families as possible. I forged an immediate bond with my Horizon editor, Amanda, whose guidance and patience were paramount when I began this process. Her insight to lobby for a full-color book has led to this beautifully finished product. The colorful images that the talented Sara Stanley created will make all the difference in the world to readers. My copyeditor, Leigh, graciously went above and beyond to ensure all the images and icons were placed correctly. Under Jeff's guidance, the Neuwirth & Associates team knocked it out of the park with the book design. And John with Horizon made our marketing calls feel like a mini pep rally.

This book became a reality only because of the outstanding team we have at Infinite Health, PLLC, current and past: Deb, Isabella, Lauren, Chloe, Angel, Katherine, Jennifer, Tim, Darrell, Andy, Braden, and Brendan. Each of them brings their unique gifts so we are able to serve hundreds of children each year. A special thanks to Jennifer, who took a jumbled stack of writing and walked me right through my writer's block.

Thank you to the great friends I have from every phase of my life. Kathy, Becky, and Wendy, and all the Random House Girls from our undergrad days at Miami University, who keep me feeling like I'm mentally twenty-one. My medical school friends, who kept me laughing through our four years together. My residency friends, who became my family and will always hold a sacred place in my heart. My yoga friends—what can I say?—they helped me see the world through a different lens.

Professionally, many brilliant people have mentored me and have touched my life deeply. My high school biology teacher, Mr. Hunt, taught my favorite science classes. Dr. John Stang's caring approach to medical student education was over-the-top incredible. Rest in peace, Dr. Stang. Cheryl Courtlandt, MD, and Amina Ahmed, MD, were great role models during residency.

Russ Greenfield, MD, and Shirley Houston, MD, are the father and mother of integrative medicine here in Charlotte, and both of them provided me with mentorship. Russ ultimately led me to the Andrew Weil Integrative Medical Fellowship, which changed my life forever.

I must mention the phenomenal integrative community here in Charlotte. We have a robust community of practitioners that has always kept me going. I send an extra dose of gratitude to my inner circle of health coaches, who created the delicious recipes in section III: the amazing sisters, Adri Warrick and Carolyn Hallett, as well as the one-of-a-kind Haynes Paschall. I have such admiration for the way all three of these women courageously continue to advocate for the health of children and families.

And lastly, thank you to Paul Smolen, MD (Docsmo). He has been a supportive figure for me over the past ten-plus years and has helped me realize it is okay to speak up about the powerful role nutrition plays in children's health.

notes

INTRODUCTION

1. Davis, K., et al. "Mirror, Mirror on the Wall, 2014." Update: "How the U.S. Health Care System Compares Internationally." *The Commonwealth Fund*. June 2014. Accessed Feb 13, 2016. http://www.commonwealthfund.org/publications /fund-reports/2014/jun/mirror-mirror.

2. Davis, K., et al. "Mirror, Mirror on the Wall, 2014."

3. Davis, K., et al. "Mirror, Mirror on the Wall, 2014."

4. OECD (2015), *Health at a Glance 2015: OECD Indicators*, OECD Publishing, Paris. Accessed February 13, 2016. doi: 10.1787/health_glance-2015-en.

CHAPTER 1

1. Zahran, H. S., et al. "Vital Signs: Asthma in Children—United States, 2001–2016." *Morbidity and Mortality Weekly Report* 67, no. 5 (2018): 149–155. doi:10.15585/mmwr.mm6705e1.

2. Silverberg, J. I., and Simpson, E. L. "Associations of Childhood Eczema Severity: A US Population-Based Study." *Dermatitis* 25, no. 3 (2014): 107–114. doi:10.1097 /DER.0000000000000034.

3. Teele, D. W., et al. "Greater Boston Otitis Media Study Group. Epidemiology of Otitis Media During the First Seven Years of Life in Children in Greater Boston: A Prospective, Cohort Study." *Journal of Infectious Diseases* 160, no. 1 (1989): 83–94. doi:10.1093/infdis/160.1.83.

4. Taylor-Black, S. A., et al. "Prevalence of Food Allergy in New York City School Children." *Annals of Allergy, Asthma & Immunology* 112, no. 6 (2014): 554–556. doi:10.1016/j.anai.2014.03.020.

5. Hill, I. D., et al. "NASPGHAN Clinical Report on the Diagnosis and Treatment of Gluten-related Disorders." *Journal of Pediatric Gastroenterology and Nutrition* 63, no. 1 (July 2016): 156–65. doi: 10.1097/MPG.0000000000001216.

6. Childhood Obesity Facts. Centers for Disease Control and Prevention. https:// www.cdc.gov/obesity/data/childhood.html. Published June 24, 2019.

7. Currie, J., Stabile, M., "Mental Health in Childhood and Human Capital." *National Bureau of Economic Research*. Working Paper 13217. https://www.nber .org/papers/w13217.pdf.

8. Lebwhohl, B., et al. "Mucosal Healing and Risk for Lymphoproliferative Malignancy in Celiac Disease. A Population-based Cohort Study." *Annals of Internal Medicine* 159, no. 3 (2013): 169–175.

9. Lebwhohl, B., et al. "Mucosal Healing and Risk for Lymphoproliferative Malignancy in Celiac Disease."

10. Lebwhohl, B., et al. "Mucosal Healing and Risk for Lymphoproliferative Malignancy in Celiac Disease."

11. Dolinoy, D. J., et al. "Epigenetic Gene Regulation: Linking Early Developmental Environment to Adult Disease." *Reproductive Toxicology* 23, no. 3 (April 2007): 297–307. https://doi.org/10.1016/j.reprotox.2006.08.012.

12. Jirtle, Randy L., et al. "Environmental Epigenomics and Disease Susceptibility." *Nature Reviews Genetics* 8, no. 4 (April 2007): 253–62. https://doi.org/10.1038/nrg2045.

13. Waterland, Robert A., and Randy L. Jirtle. "Transposable Elements: Targets for Early Nutritional Effects on Epigenetic Gene Regulation." *Molecular and Cellular Biology* 23, no. 15 (August 1, 2003): 5293–5300. https://doi.org/10.1128/MCB.23.15.5293-5300.2003.

CHAPTER 2

1. Castro-Rodrigues, J. A., et al. "A Clinical Index to Define Risk of Asthma in Young Children with Recurrent Wheezing." *Am J Respir Crit Care Med* 162, no. 4 part 1 (October 2000): 1403–1406. Accessed February 15, 2016. 10.1164/ajrccm.162.4.9912111.

CHAPTER 3

1. Hijazi Z., et al. "Intestinal Permeability Is Increased in Bronchial Asthma." *Arch Dis Child* 89 (2004): 227–229.

2. "5 Things to Know About Triclosan." U.S. Food & Drug Administration. May 16, 2019. https://www.fda.gov/consumers/consumer-updates/5-things-know-about-triclosan.

3. Okada, H., et al. "The 'hygiene hypothesis' for autoimmune and allergic diseases: an update." *Clin Exp Immunol* 160, no. 1 (2010): 1–9. doi: 10.1111/j.1365-2249.2010.04139.x.

4. Benbrook, C. "Trends in Glyphosate Herbicide Use in the United States and Globally." *Environ Scie Eur* 28, no. 3 (2016). https://doi.org/10.1186/s12302-016-0070-0.

5. "Outpatient Antibiotic Prescriptions—United States, 2015." Centers for Disease Control and Prevention. Accessed Jan. 25, 2018. https://www.cdc.gov/antibiotic-use/community/pdfs/Annual-report-2015.pdf.

6. National Research Council (U.S.) Committee to Study the Human Health Effects of Subtherapeutic Antibiotic Use in Animal Feeds. *The Effects on Human Health of Subtherapeutic Use of Antimicrobials in Animal Feeds.* Washington (D.C.): National Academies Press (U.S.), 1980. Appendix K, Antibiotics In Animal Feeds. Available from https://www.ncbi.nlm.nih.gov/books/NBK216502/.

7. Bowen, Alison. "1 in 3 U.S. Women Have C-sections. How Chicago Doctors Are Working to Change That." *Chicago Tribune.* May 15, 2017. https://www.

chicagotribune.com/lifestyles/health/ct-cesarean-sections-births-health-0515
-20170515-story.html.

8. Fassano, A. "Leaky Gut and Autoimmune Diseases." *Clin Rev Allergy Immunol* 42,
    no. 1 (February 2012): 71–78. Accessed March 16, 2016. doi: 10.1007/s12016
    -011-8291-x.

9. Fassano, A. "Leaky Gut and Autoimmune Diseases."

CHAPTER 4

1. Sanchez, Albert, et al. "Role of Sugars in Human Neutrophilic Phagocytosis." *The
    American Journal of Clinical Nutrition* 26, no. 11 (November 1, 1973): 1180–1184.
    https://doi.org/10.1093/ajcn/26.11.1180.

2. Di Costanzo, Margherita, and Roberto Berni Canani. "Lactose Intolerance:
    Common Misunderstandings." *Annals of Nutrition and Metabolism* 73, no. Suppl. 4
    (2018): 30–37. https://doi.org/10.1159/000493669.

3. Di Costanzo, Margherita, and Roberto Berni Canani. "Lactose Intolerance:
    Common Misunderstandings."

4. "Celiac Disease Facts and Figures." Celiac Disease Center, The University of
    Chicago Medicine. https://www.cureceliacdisease.org/wp-content/uploads/341
    _CDCFactSheets8_FactsFigures.pdf.

5. "Celiac Disease Facts and Figures."

6. Di Costanzo, Margherita, and Roberto Berni Canani. "Lactose Intolerance:
    Common Misunderstandings."

CHAPTER 5

1. Sengar, G., Sharma, H. K. "Food Caramels: A Review." *J Food Sci Technol* 51, no. 9
    (2012): 1686–1696. doi: 10.1007/s13197-012-0633-z.

2. Akbaraly, Tasnime N., et al. "Alternative Healthy Eating Index and Mortality
    over 18 Years of Follow-up: Results from the Whitehall II Cohort." *The American
    Journal of Clinical Nutrition* 94, no. 1 (July 1, 2011): 247–53. https://doi
    .org/10.3945/ajcn.111.013128.

3. Belin, Rashad J., et al. "Diet Quality and the Risk of Cardiovascular Disease: The
    Women's Health Initiative (WHI)." *The American Journal of Clinical Nutrition* 94,
    no. 1 (July 1, 2011): 49–57. https://doi.org/10.3945/ajcn.110.011221.

4. Fryar, Cheryl D., et al. "Prevalence of Overweight, Obesity, and Severe Obesity
    Among Children and Adolescents Aged 2–19 Years: United States, 1963–1965
    Through 2015–2016." National Center for Health Statistics. September 2018.
    https://www.cdc.gov/nchs/data/hestat/obesity_child_15_16/obesity_child_15_16
    .htm.

5. "Get the Facts: Sugar-Sweetened Beverages and Consumption." Centers for
    Disease Control and Prevention. November 18, 2020. https://www.cdc.gov
    /nutrition/data-statistics/sugar-sweetened-beverages-intake.html.

6. Sanchez, Albert, et al. "Role of Sugars in Human Neutrophilic Phagocytosis." *The
    American Journal of Clinical Nutrition* 26, no. 11 (November 1, 1973): 1180–84.
    https://doi.org/10.1093/ajcn/26.11.1180.

7. Jastreboff, Ania, et al. "Altered Brain Response to Drinking Glucose and Fructose in Obese Adolescents." *Diabetes* 65, no. 7 (July 2016): 1929–39. https://doi .org/10.2337/db15-1216.

8. Beilharz, Jessica, et al. "Diet-Induced Cognitive Deficits: The Role of Fat and Sugar, Potential Mechanisms and Nutritional Interventions." *Nutrients* 7, no. 8 (August 12, 2015): 6719–38. https://doi.org/10.3390/nu7085307.

9. Ward, Zachary J., et al. "Simulation of Growth Trajectories of Childhood Obesity into Adulthood." *New England Journal of Medicine* 377, no. 22 (November 30, 2017): 2145–53. https://doi.org/10.1056/NEJMoa1703860.

10. Ruiz-Ojeda, Francisco Javier, et al. "Effects of Sweeteners on the Gut Microbiota: A Review of Experimental Studies and Clinical Trials." *Advances in Nutrition* 10, suppl. 1 (January 1, 2019): S31–48. https://doi.org/10.1093/advances/nmy037.

11. Micha, Renata, et al. "Processing of Meats and Cardiovascular Risk: Time to Focus on Preservatives." *BMC Medicine* 11, no. 1 (December 2013): 136. https:// doi.org/10.1186/1741.

12. Micha, Renata, et al. "Unprocessed Red and Processed Meats and Risk of Coronary Artery Disease and Type 2 Diabetes—An Updated Review of the Evidence." *Current Atherosclerosis Reports* 14, no. 6 (December 2012): 515–24. https://doi.org/10.1007/s11883-012-0282-8.

13. Rohrmann, Sabine, et al. "Meat Consumption and Mortality—Results from the European Prospective Investigation into Cancer and Nutrition." *BMC Medicine* 11, no. 1 (December 2013): 63. https://doi.org/10.1186/1741-7015-11-63.

14. Crowe, William, et al. "A Review of the In Vivo Evidence Investigating the Role of Nitrite Exposure from Processed Meat Consumption in the Development of Colorectal Cancer." *Nutrients* 11, no. 11 (November 5, 2019): 2673. https://doi .org/10.3390/nu11112673.

15. Kleinbongard, Petra, et al. "Plasma Nitrite Concentrations Reflect the Degree of Endothelial Dysfunction in Humans." *Free Radical Biology and Medicine* 40, no. 2 (January 2006): 295–302. https://doi.org/10.1016/j.freeradbiomed.2005.08.025.

CHAPTER 6

1. Mickleborough, T. D., Lindley, M. R., Lonescu, A. A., and Fly, A. D., "Protective Effect of Fish Oil Supplementation on Exercise-induced Bronchoconstriction in Asthma." *Chest* 129 (2006): 39–49.

2. Simopoulos, A. P. "Human Requirement for N-3 Polyunsaturated Fatty Acids." *Poult Sci* 79, no. 7 (July 2000): 961–970. Accessed February 14, 2016. http:// ps.oxfordjournals.org/content/79/7/961.long.

3. Haag M., "Essential Fatty Acids and the Brain." *Revue Canadienne de Psychiatrie* 48, no. 3 (2003):195–203.

4. Chang, Chia-Yu, et al. "Essential Fatty Acids and Human Brain." *Acta Neurol Taiwan* 18, no. 4 (December 2009): 231–241.

5. Makki, Kassem, et al. "The Impact of Dietary Fiber on Gut Microbiota in Host Health and Disease." *Cell Host & Microbe* 23, no. 6 (June 2018): 705–15. https:// doi.org/10.1016/j.chom.2018.05.012.

6. Makki, Kassem, et al. "The Impact of Dietary Fiber on Gut Microbiota in Host Health and Disease."

7. McDonald, Daniel, et al. "American Gut: An Open Platform for Citizen Science Microbiome Research." Edited by Casey S. Greene. *MSystems* 3, no. 3 (May 15, 2018): e00031-18, /msystems/3/3/msys.00031-18.atom. https://doi.org/10.1128/mSystems.00031-18.

8. Gupta, Charu, and Dhan Prakash. "Phytonutrients as Therapeutic Agents." *Journal of Complementary and Integrative Medicine* 11, no. 3 (January 1, 2014). https://doi.org/10.1515/jcim-2013-0021.

9. Simopoulos, A. P. and Salem, N. Jr. "n−3 Fatty Acids in Eggs from Range-fed Greek Chickens." *New England Journal of Medicine* 321 (1989): 1412–1415.

10. Kris-Etherton, P. M., et al. "Polyunsaturated Fatty Acids in the Food Chain in the United States." *Am J Clin Nutr* 71, no. 1 (January 2000): 179S–188S. Accessed February 14, 1016. http://ajcn.nutrition.org/content/71/1/179S.full?ijkey=5c7af875f3dc71a303f7df78c52145e8b7c31643.

CHAPTER 7

1. "Got Milk Article." Originally published in *UC Davis Innovator*, Spring 1999. Reprinted at https://milk.com/value/innovator-spring99.html.

2. "Got Milk Article."

3. "Got Milk Article."

4. Physicians Committee for Responsible Medicine and Catherine Holmes for herself and as a representative for others similarly situated (Plaintiff) versus Kraft Foods, Inc., General Mills, inc., Dannon Company, Inc, McNeil P.P.C., Inc., International Dairy Foods Association, Dairy Management, Inc., National Dairy Council, and Lifeway Foods, Inc. (Defendants). https://milk.procon.org/wp-content/uploads/sites/44/pcrmlawsuit.pdf.

5. Keast, D. R., et al. "Food Sources of Energy and Nutrients among Children in the United States: National Health and Nutrition Examination Survey 2003–2006." *Nutrients* 5, no. 1 (2013): 283–301.

6. Hegsted, D. M. "Calcium and Osteoporosis." *The Journal of Nutrition* 116, no. 11 (November 1, 1986): 2316–19. https://doi.org/10.1093/jn/116.11.2316.

7. Hegsted, D. Mark , Calcium, and the Modern Diet." *The American Journal of Clinical Nutrition* 74, no. 5 (November 1, 2001): 571–73. https://doi.org/10.1093/ajcn/74.5.571.

8. Feskanich, D., et al. "Milk, Dietary Calcium, and Bone Fractures in Women: A 12-Year Prospective Study." *American Journal of Public Health* 87, no. 6 (June 1997): 992–97. https://doi.org/10.2105/AJPH.87.6.992.

9. Hunt, Curtiss D., and LuAnn K. Johnson. "Calcium Requirements: New Estimations for Men and Women by Cross-Sectional Statistical Analyses of Calcium Balance Data from Metabolic Studies." *The American Journal of Clinical Nutrition* 86, no. 4 (October 1, 2007): 1054–63. https://doi.org/10.1093/ajcn/86.4.1054.

10. Ross, A. Catharine, et al. "The 2011 Report on Dietary Reference Intakes for Calcium and Vitamin D from the Institute of Medicine: What Clinicians Need to Know." *The Journal of Clinical Endocrinology & Metabolism* 96, no. 1 (January 2011): 53–58. https://doi.org/10.1210/jc.2010-2704.

11. "Nutrition and Bone Health: With Particular Reference to Calcium and Vitamin D. Report of the Subgroup on Bone Health, Working Group on the Nutritional

Status of the Population of the Committee on Medical Aspects of the Food Nutrition Policy." *Reports on Health and Social Subjects* 49 (1998): iii–xvii, 1–24.

12.　Katz, David. "Vitamin D and Calcium: Is the IOM Right to Recommend We Get Less?" Huffington Post. May 25, 2011. https://www.huffpost.com/entry /vitamind--andcalcium-shouldwe--becautious_b_789842.

13.　Feskanich, Diane, et al. "Milk Consumption During Teenage Years and Risk of Hip Fractures in Older Adults." *JAMA Pediatrics* 168, no. 1 (January 1, 2014): 54. https://doi.org/10.1001/jamapediatrics.2013.3821.

14.　"Calcium." The Nutrition Source, T. H. Chan School of Public Health, Harvard University. n.d. http://www.hsph.harvard.edu/nutritionsource/calcium-full-story/.

15.　Weaver, C. M., et al. "The National Osteoporosis Foundation's Position Statement on Peak Bone Mass Development and Lifestyle Factors: A Systematic Review and Implementation Recommendations." *Osteoporosis International* 27, no. 4 (April 2016): 1281–1386. https://doi.org/10.1007/s00198-015-3440-3.

16.　Feskanich, Diane, et al. "Milk Consumption During Teenage Years and Risk of Hip Fractures in Older Adults."

17.　Palacios, Cristina. "The Role of Nutrients in Bone Health, from A to Z." *Critical Reviews in Food Science and Nutrition* 46, no. 8 (December 2006): 621–28. https://doi.org/10.1080/10408390500466174.

18.　Ismail, Adel A. A., and Nour A. Ismail. "Magnesium: A Mineral Essential for Health Yet Generally Underestimated or Even Ignored." *Journal of Nutrition & Food Sciences* 6, no. 4 (2016). https://doi.org/10.4172/2155-9600.1000523.

19.　Rosanoff, Andrea, et al. "Suboptimal Magnesium Status in the United States: Are the Health Consequences Underestimated?" *Nutrition Reviews* 70, no. 3 (March 2012): 153–64. https://doi.org/10.1111/j.1753-4887.2011.00465.x.

20.　Abrams, Steven A., et al. "Magnesium Metabolism in 4-Year-Old to 8-Year-Old Children." *Journal of Bone and Mineral Research* 29, no. 1 (January 2014): 118–22. https://doi.org/10.1002/jbmr.2021.

21.　Feskanich, Diane, et al. "Milk Consumption During Teenage Years and Risk of Hip Fractures in Older Adults."

22.　Winzenberg, Tania M, et al. "Calcium Supplementation for Improving Bone Mineral Density in Children." Edited by Cochrane Musculoskeletal Group. *Cochrane Database of Systematic Reviews*, April 19, 2006. https://doi.org /10.1002/14651858.CD005119.pub2.

23.　Merrilees, M. J., et al. "Effects of Dairy Food Supplements on Bone Mineral Density in Teenage Girls." *European Journal of Nutrition* 39, no. 6 (December 1, 2000): 256–62. https://doi.org/10.1007/s003940070004.

24.　Lee, W. T. K., et al. "A Follow-up Study on the Effects of Calcium-Supplement Withdrawal and Puberty on Bone Acquisition of Children." *The American Journal of Clinical Nutrition* 64, no. 1 (July 1, 1996): 71–77. https://doi.org/10.1093 /ajcn/64.1.71.

25.　Lee, W. T. K., et al. "Bone Mineral Acquisition in Low Calcium Intake Children Following the Withdrawal of Calcium Supplement." *Acta Paediatrica* 86, no. 6 (June 1997): 570–76. https://doi.org/10.1111/j.1651-2227.1997.tb08936.x.

26.　Slemenda, Charles W., et al. "Reduced Rates of Skeletal Remodeling Are Associated with Increased Bone Mineral Density During the Development of

Peak Skeletal Mass." *Journal of Bone and Mineral Research* 12, no. 4 (April 1, 1997): 676–82. https://doi.org/10.1359/jbmr.1997.12.4.676.

27. Abrams, Steven A., et al. "Magnesium Metabolism in 4-Year-Old to 8-Year-Old Children."

28. Abrams, Steven A, et al. "Pubertal Girls Only Partially Adapt to Low Dietary Calcium Intakes." *Journal of Bone and Mineral Research* 19, no. 5 (January 19, 2004): 759–63. https://doi.org/10.1359/jbmr.040122.

29. Feskanich, Diane, et al. "Milk Consumption During Teenage Years and Risk of Hip Fractures in Older Adults."

30. Weaver, C. M., et al. "The National Osteoporosis Foundation's Position Statement on Peak Bone Mass Development and Lifestyle Factors: A Systematic Review and Implementation Recommendations." *Osteoporosis International* 27, no. 4 (April 2016): 1281–1386. https://doi.org/10.1007/s00198-015-3440-3.

31. Weaver, C. M., et al. "The National Osteoporosis Foundation's Position Statement on Peak Bone Mass Development and Lifestyle Factors."

32. Dr. Oski was the Chairman of Pediatrics at Johns Hopkins School of Medicine, one of the premier pediatric hospitals in the country. He also wrote many of the textbooks used to train pediatricians around the globe.

33. Novembre, E., and A. Vierucci. "Milk Allergy/Intolerance and Atopic Dermatitis in Infancy and Childhood." *Allergy* 56 Suppl. 67 (2001): 105–8. https://doi .org/10.1111/j.1398-9995.2001.00931.x.

34. Sloper, K. S., et al. "Children with Atopic Eczema. I: Clinical Response to Food Elimination and Subsequent Double-Blind Food Challenge." *QJM: An International Journal of Medicine* 80, no. 2 (August 1991): 677–693, https://doi .org/10.1093/oxfordjournals.qjmed.a068619.

35. Ress, Krista, et al. "Celiac Disease in Children with Atopic Dermatitis." *Pediatric Dermatology* 31, no. 4 (July 2014): 483–88. https://doi.org/10.1111/pde.12372.

36. Leyden, James J., et al. "Staphylococcus Aureus in the Lesions of Atopic Dermatitis." *British Journal of Dermatology* 90, no. 5 (May 1974): 525. https://doi. org/10.1111/j.1365-2133.1974.tb06447.x.

37. Nsouli, T. M., et al. "Role of Food Allergy in Serous Otitis Media." *Annals of Allergy* 73, no. 3 (September 1994): 215–19.

38. Iacono, Giuseppe, et al. "Intolerance of Cow's Milk and Chronic Constipation in Children." *New England Journal of Medicine* 339, no. 16 (October 15, 1998): 1100–1104. https://doi.org/10.1056/NEJM199810153391602.

39. Murray, M. G., et al. "Milk-Induced Wheezing in Children with Asthma." *Allergologia et Immunopathologia* 41, no. 5 (September 2013): 310–14. https://doi .org/10.1016/j.aller.2012.07.002.

40. Yusoff, Noor Aini Mohd, et al. "The Effects of Exclusion of Dietary Egg and Milk in the Management of Asthmatic Children: A Pilot Study." *Journal of the Royal Society for the Promotion of Health* 124, no. 2 (March 2004): 74–80. https://doi .org/10.1177/146642400412400211.

41. Høst, A., and S. Halken. "The Role of Allergy in Childhood Asthma." *Allergy* 55, no. 7 (July 2000): 600–608. https://doi.org/10.1034/j.1398-9995.2000.00122.x.

42. Murray, M. G., et al. "Milk-Induced Wheezing in Children with Asthma." *Allergologia et Immunopathologia* 41, no. 5 (September 2013): 310–14. https://doi .org/10.1016/j.aller.2012.07.002.

43. Iacono, G., et al. "Gastroesophageal Reflux and Cow's Milk Allergy in Infants: A Prospective Study." J of Allergy and Clin Immunol 97, no. 3 (1996): 822–827. Accessed February 16, 2016. doi: 10.1016/S0091-6749(96)80160-6.

44. Farahmand, F., et al. "Cow's Milk Allergy Among Children with Gastroesophageal Reflux Disease." *Gut Liver* 5, no. 3 (September 2011): 298–301. Accessed February 16, 2016. doi:10.5009/gnl.2011.5.3.298.

45. Jakobsson, I., and T. Lindberg. "Cow's Milk Proteins Cause Infantile Colic in Breast-Fed Infants: A Double-Blind Crossover Study." *Pediatrics* 71, no. 2 (February 1983): 268–71.

46. Ziegler, Ekhard E. "Consumption of Cow's Milk as a Cause of Iron Deficiency in Infants and Toddlers." *Nutrition Reviews* 69 (November 2011): S37–42. https:// doi.org/10.1111/j.1753-4887.2011.00431.x.

CHAPTER 8

1. "Children Eating More Fruit, but Fruit and Vegetable Intake Still Too Low." Centers for Disease Control and Prevention. August 5, 2014. https://www.cdc .gov/media/releases/2014/p0805-fruits-vegetables.html.

2. "Children Eating More Fruit, but Fruit and Vegetable Intake Still Too Low."

3. Davis, Donald R., Melvin D. Epp, and Hugh D. Riordan. "Changes in USDA Food Composition Data for 43 Garden Crops, 1950 to 1999." *Journal of the American College of Nutrition* 23, no. 6 (December 2004): 669–82. https://doi.org/10.1080 /07315724.2004.10719409.

4. "Food Consumption, 2020." Centers for Disease Control and Prevention. February 5, 2021. https://www.cdc.gov/nchs/products/visual-gallery/fast-food -consumption.htm?Sort=Title%3A%3Aasc.

5. "Fast Food Consumption Among Adults in the United States, 2013–2016." NCCHS Dta Brief no. 322. National Center for Health Statistics. October 2018. https://www.cdc.gov/nchs/products/databriefs/db322.htm#:~:text=In%20 2013%E2%80%932016%2C%2036.6%25,adults%20aged%2060%20and%20 over.

6. Research Findings #21: Health Care Expenses in the United States, 2000. Agency for Healthcare Research and Quality, Rockville, MD. April 2004. http://www .Meps.Ahrq.Gov/Data_files/Publications/Rf21/Rf21.Shtml.

CHAPTER 10

1. Kuiper, G. G., et al. "Interaction of Estrogenic Chemicals and Phytoestrogens with Estrogen Receptor." *Endocrinology* 139 (1998): 4252–4263.

2. Dickerson S.M., and Gore, A. C. "Estrogenic Environmental Endocrine-disrupting Chemical Effects on Reproductive Neuroendocrine Function and Dysfunction Across the Life Cycle." *Rev Endocr Metab Disord* 8 (2007): 143–159.

3. Cao, Y., et al. "Isoflavones in Urine, Saliva and Blood of Infants—Data From a Pilot Study on the Estrogenic Activity of Soy Formula." *J Expo Sci Environ Epidemiol* 19 (2009): 223–234.

4. Calafat, A. M., and Needham, L. L. "Human Exposures and Body Burdens of Endocrine-disrupting Chemicals." In Gore, A. C., ed. *Endocrine-disrupting chemicals: from basic research to clinical practice* (Totowa, NJ: Humana Press: 2007): 253–268.

SECTION II

1. McDonald, Daniel, et al. "American Gut: An Open Platform for Citizen Science Microbiome Research." Edited by Casey S. Greene. *MSystems* 3, no. 3 (May 15, 2018): e00031-18, /msystems/3/3/msys.00031-18.atom. https://doi.org/10.1128/mSystems.00031-18.

2. Griffin, S. M., D. Alderson, and J. R. Farndon. "Acid Resistant Lipase as Replacement Therapy in Chronic Pancreatic Exocrine Insufficiency: A Study in Dogs." *Gut* 30, no. 7 (July 1, 1989): 1012–15. https://doi.org/10.1136/gut.30.7.1012.

3. Lim, Stephen S., et al. "A Comparative Risk Assessment of Burden of Disease and Injury Attributable to 67 Risk Factors and Risk Factor Clusters in 21 Regions, 1990–2010: A Systematic Analysis for the Global Burden of Disease Study 2010." *The Lancet* 380, no. 9859 (December 2012): 2224–60. https://doi.org/10.1016/S0140-6736(12)61766-8.

4. Stevens, L. J., et al. "Essential Fatty Acid Metabolism in Boys with Attention-Deficit Hyperactivity Disorder." *The American Journal of Clinical Nutrition* 62, no. 4 (October 1, 1995): 761–68. https://doi.org/10.1093/ajcn/62.4.761.

5. Chang, Chia-Yu, et al. "Essential Fatty Acids and Human Brain."

6. Haag M., "Essential Fatty Acids and the Brain."

7. Shapiro, et al. "Emerging Risk Factors for Postpartum Depression: Serotonin Transporter Genotype and Omega-3 Fatty Acid Status." *Can J Psychiatry* 57, no. 11 (November 2012): 704–12.

8. Forrest, Kimberly Y. Z., et al. "Prevalence and Correlates of Vitamin D Deficiency in US Adults." *Nutrition Research* 31, no. 1 (January 2011): 48–54. https://doi.org/10.1016/j.nutres.2010.12.001.

9. Sahota, O. "Understanding Vitamin D Deficiency." *Age and Ageing* 43, no. 5 (September 1, 2014): 589–91. https://doi.org/10.1093/ageing/afu104.

10. Rosanoff, Andrea, et al. "Suboptimal Magnesium Status in the United States: Are the Health Consequences Underestimated?" *Nutrition Reviews* 70, no. 3 (March 2012): 153–64. https://doi.org/10.1111/j.1753-4887.2011.00465.x.

11. Sandstead, H. H. "Understanding Zinc: Recent Observations and Interpretations." *The Journal of Laboratory and Clinical Medicine* 124, no. 3 (September 1994): 322–27.

12. Heyneman, Catherine A. "Zinc Deficiency and Taste Disorders." *Annals of Pharmacotherapy* 30, no. 2 (February 1996): 186–87. https://doi.org/10.1177/106002809603000215.

13. Black, M. M. "Zinc Deficiency and Child Development." *The American Journal of Clinical Nutrition* 68, no. 2 (August 1, 1998): 464S–469S. https://doi.org/10.1093/ajcn/68.2.464S.

14. Solomons, Noel W. "Mild Human Zinc Deficiency Produces an Imbalance Between Cell-Mediated and Humoral Immunity." *Nutrition Reviews* 56, no. 1 (April 27, 2009): 27–28. https://doi.org/10.1111/j.1753-4887.1998.tb01656.x.

15. Lazzerini, Marzia, and Humphrey Wanzira. "Oral Zinc for Treating Diarrhoea in Children." Edited by Cochrane Infectious Diseases Group. *Cochrane Database of Systematic Reviews*, December 20, 2016. https://doi.org/10.1002/14651858 .CD005436.pub5.

16. "PMNCH Knowledge Summary 18—Nutrition." The Partnership for Maternal, Newborn, and Child Health. 2012 edition. Accessed at https://cdn2.sph.harvard .edu/wp-content/uploads/sites/32/2017/05/ks18.pdf.

17. Infusino, Fabio, et al. "Diet Supplementation, Probiotics, and Nutraceuticals in SARS-CoV-2 Infection: A Scoping Review." *Nutrients* 12, no. 6 (June 8, 2020): 1718. https://doi.org/10.3390/nu12061718.

18. Filgueiras, M. S., et al. "Vitamin D Status, Oxidative Stress, and Inflammation in Children and Adolescents: A Systematic Review." *Critical Reviews in Food Science and Nutrition* 60, no. 4 (February 21, 2020): 660–69. https://doi.org/10.1080/104 08398.2018.1546671.

APPENDIX

1. Löfmark, et al, 2006. "Prolonged impact of a one-week course of clindamycin on Enterococcus spp. in human normal microbiota." *Infectious Diseases* 41, no. 3 (2009): 215–219. doi: 10.1080/00365540802651897.

2. Mcburney, W. T. "Perturbation of the enterobacterial microflora detected by molecular analysis." *Microbial Ecology in Health and Disease* 11, no. 3 (1999): 175–179. doi: 10.1080/089106099435763.

3. Vanderhoof, J. A., and R. J. Young. "Probiotics in Pediatrics." *Pediatrics* 109, no. 5 (May 1, 2002): 956–58. https://doi.org/10.1542/peds.109.5.956.

4. Johnson, Rachel K., et al. "Dietary Sugars Intake and Cardiovascular Health: A Scientific Statement From the American Heart Association." *Circulation* 120, no. 11 (September 15, 2009): 1011–20. https://doi.org/10.1161/CIRCULATIONAHA .109.192627.

5. "Usual Intake of Added Sugars." National Cancer Institute. *Usual Dietary Intakes: Food Intakes, U.S. Population 2001–04*. November 2008. Accessed February 20, 2016. http://riskfactor.cancer.gov/diet/usualintakes/pop/ t35.html.

6. Jianqin, Sun, et al. "Effects of Milk Containing Only A2 Beta Casein versus Milk Containing Both A1 and A2 Beta Casein Proteins on Gastrointestinal Physiology, Symptoms of Discomfort, and Cognitive Behavior of People with Self-Reported Intolerance to Traditional Cows' Milk." *Nutrition Journal* 15, no. 1 (December 2015): 35. https://doi.org/10.1186/s12937-016-0147-z.

7. Institute of Medicine, Food and Nutrition Board. *Dietary Reference Intakes for Calcium and Vitamin D* (Washington, DC: National Academy Press, 2010). https://ods.od.nih.gov/factsheets/VitaminD-HealthProfessional/#en1.

8. Ahrens, Katherine A., et al. "Adherence to Vitamin D Recommendations Among U.S. Infants Aged 0 to 11 Months, NHANES, 2009 to 2012." *Clinical Pediatrics* 55, no. 6 (June 2016): 555–56. https://doi.org/10.1177/0009922815589916.

9. Lu, Z., et al. "An Evaluation of the Vitamin D3 Content in Fish: Is the Vitamin D Content Adequate to Satisfy the Dietary Requirement for Vitamin D?" *The Journal of Steroid Biochemistry and Molecular Biology* 103, no. 3–5 (March 2007): 642–44. https://doi.org/10.1016/j.jsbmb.2006.12.010.

further reading

FACTORS THAT IMPAIR DIGESTION AND DIGESTIVE ENZYME FUNCTION

Alenina, Natalia, and Friederike Klempin. "The Role of Serotonin in Adult Hippocampal Neurogenesis." *Behavioural Brain Research* 277 (January 2015): 49–57. https://doi.org/10.1016/j.bbr.2014.07.038.

Griffin, S. M., D. Alderson, and J. R. Farndon. "Acid Resistant Lipase as Replacement Therapy in Chronic Pancreatic Exocrine Insufficiency: A Study in Dogs." *Gut* 30, no. 7 (July 1, 1989): 1012–15. https://doi.org/10.1136/gut.30.7.1012.

Ido, Hiroki, et al. "Combination of Gluten-Digesting Enzymes Improved Symptoms of Non-Celiac Gluten Sensitivity: A Randomized Single-Blind, Placebo-Controlled Crossover Study." *Clinical and Translational Gastroenterology* 9, no. 9 (September 2018): e181. https://doi.org/10.1038/s41424-018-0052-1.

Mitea, C. R., et al. "Efficient Degradation of Gluten by a Prolyl Endoprotease in a Gastrointestinal Model: Implications for Coeliac Disease." *Gut* 57, no. 1 (May 14, 2007): 25–32. https://doi.org/10.1136/gut.2006.111609.

Money, M. E., et al. "Pilot Study: A Randomised, Double Blind, Placebo Controlled Trial of Pancrealipase for the Treatment of Postprandial Irritable Bowel Syndrome-Diarrhoea." *Frontline Gastroenterology* 2, no. 1 (January 1, 2011): 48–56. https://doi.org/10.1136/fg.2010.002253.

O'Mahony, S.M., et al. "Serotonin, Tryptophan Metabolism and the Brain-Gut-Microbiome Axis." *Behavioural Brain Research* 277 (January 2015): 32–48. https://doi.org/10.1016/j.bbr.2014.07.027.

Roxas, Mario. "The Role of Enzyme Supplementation in Digestive Disorders." *Alternative Medicine Review: A Journal of Clinical Therapeutic* 13, no. 4 (December 2008): 307–14.

Singer, Sanford, et al. "Pancreatic Enzyme Supplementation in Patients with Atopic Dermatitis and Food Allergies: An Open-Label Pilot Study." *Pediatric Drugs* 21, no. 1 (February 2019): 41–45. https://doi.org/10.1007/s40272-018-0321-1.

Walther, Barbara, et al. "GutSelf: Interindividual Variability in the Processing of Dietary Compounds by the Human Gastrointestinal Tract." *Molecular Nutrition & Food Research* 63, no. 21 (November 2019): 1900677. https://doi.org/10.1002/mnfr.201900677.

Widodo, Ariani Dewi, et al. "Pancreatic Enzyme Replacement Therapy (PERT) in Children with Persistent Diarrhea: Avoidance of Elemental Diet Need, Accessibility and Costs." *Asia Pacific Journal of Clinical Nutrition* 27, no. 3 (2018): 512–18. https://doi .org/10.6133/apjcn.082017.05.

Wier, Heather A., and Robert J. Kuhn. "Pancreatic Enzyme Supplementation." *Current Opinion in Pediatrics* 23, no. 5 (October 2011): 541–44. https://doi.org/10.1097 /MOP.0b013e32834a1b33.

FIBER

Hijaz, N., et al. "Diet and Childhood Asthma in a Society in Transition: A Study in Urban and Rural Saudi Arabia." *Thorax* 55, no. 9 (September 2000): 775–779. Accessed March 23, 2016. doi:10.1136/thorax.55.9.775.

Makki, Kassem, et al. "The Impact of Dietary Fiber on Gut Microbiota in Host Health and Disease." *Cell Host & Microbe* 23, no. 6 (June 2018): 705–15. https://doi .org/10.1016/j.chom.2018.05.012.

McDonald, Daniel, et al. "American Gut: An Open Platform for Citizen Science Microbiome Research." Edited by Casey S. Greene. *MSystems* 3, no. 3 (May 15, 2018): e00031-18, /msystems/3/3/msys.00031-18.atom. https://doi.org/10.1128/ mSystems.00031-18.

MAGNESIUM

Ismail, A. A. A., et al. "Chronic Magnesium Deficiency and Human Disease; Time for Reappraisal?" *QJM: An International Journal of Medicine* 111, no. 11 (November 1, 2018): 759–63. https://doi.org/10.1093/qjmed/hcx186.

Ismail, Adel A. A., and Nour A. Ismail. "Magnesium: A Mineral Essential for Health Yet Generally Underestimated or Even Ignored." *Journal of Nutrition & Food Sciences* 6, no. 4 (2016). https://doi.org/10.4172/2155-9600.1000523.

Rosanoff, Andrea, et al. "Suboptimal Magnesium Status in the United States: Are the Health Consequences Underestimated?" *Nutrition Reviews* 70, no. 3 (March 2012): 153–64. https://doi.org/10.1111/j.1753-4887.2011.00465.x.

Shaikh, Mohammed Nadeem, et al. "Serum Magnesium and Vitamin D Levels as Indicators of Asthma Severity." *Pulmonary Medicine* 2016 (2016): 1–5. https://doi .org/10.1155/2016/1643717.

OMEGA-3 FATS

Chang, Chia-Yu, et al. "Essential Fatty Acids and Human Brain." *Acta Neurol Taiwan* 18, no. 4 (December 2009): 231–241.

Haag M., "Essential Fatty Acids and the Brain." *Revue Canadienne de Psychiatrie* 48, no. 3 (2003): 195–203.

Shapiro, et al. "Emerging Risk Factors for Postpartum Depression: Serotonin Transporter Genotype and Omega-3 Fatty Acid Status." *Can J Psychiatry* 57, no. 11 (November 2012): 704–12.

Simopoulos, A. P. "Human Requirement for N-3 Polyunsaturated Fatty Acids." *Poult Sci* 79, no. 7 (July 2000): 961–70. Accessed February 14, 2016. http://ps.oxfordjournals.org /content/79/7/961.long.

Sinn, N., et al. "Oiling the Brain: A Review of Randomized Controlled Trials of Omega-3 Fatty Acids in Psychopathology Across the Lifespan." *Nutrients* 2, no. 2 *(February* 2010): 128–170. Accessed February 14, 2016. doi: 10.3390/nu2020128.

Stevens, L. J., et al. "Essential Fatty Acid Metabolism in Boys with Attention-Deficit Hyperactivity Disorder."·*The American Journal of Clinical Nutrition* 62, no. 4 (October 1, 1995): 761–68. https://doi.org/10.1093/ajcn/62.4.761.

Wozniak, J., et al. "Omega-3 Fatty Acid Monotherapy for Pediatric Bipolar Disorder: A Prospective Open-label Trial." *European Neuropsychopharmacology* 17, nos. 6–7 (May 2007): 440–447. Accessed February 14, 2016. http://www.europeanneuropsychopharmacology .com/article/S0924-977X(06)00256-2/fulltext.

PROBIOTICS (SPECIFICALLY *LACTOBACILLUS PLANTARUM*)

Flórez, Ana Belén, et. al. "Susceptibility of Lactobacillus Plantarum Strains to Six Antibiotics and Definition of New Susceptibility-Resistance Cutoff Values." *Microbial Drug Resistance (Larchmont, N.Y.)* 12, no. 4 (2006)· 252–56. https://doi.org/10.1089 /mdr.2006.12.252.

Jonkers, Daisy, and Reinhold Stockbrügger. "Probiotics and Inflammatory Bowel Disease. *Journal of the Royal Society of Medicine* 96, no. 4 (April 2003): 167–71.

Klarin, Bengt, et al. "Adhesion of the Probiotic Bacterium Lactobacillus Plantarum 299v onto the Gut Mucosa in Critically Ill Patients: A Randomized Open Trial." *Critical Care* 9, no. 3 (2005): R285. https://doi.org/10.1186/cc3522.

Mangell, Peter, et al. "Adhesive Capability of Lactobacillus Plantarum 299v Is Important for Preventing Bacterial Translocation in Endotoxemic Rats." *APMIS* 114, no. 9 (September 2006): 611–18. https://doi.org/10.1111/j.1600-0463.2006.apm_369.x.

Petrof, Elaine O., et al. "Bacteria-Free Solution Derived from Lactobacillus Plantarum Inhibits Multiple NF-KappaB Pathways and Inhibits Proteasome Function." *Inflammatory Bowel Diseases* 15, no. 10 (October 2009): 1537–1547. https://doi.org/10 .1002/ibd.20930.

VITAMIN D

Filgueiras, M. S., et al. "Vitamin D Status, Oxidative Stress, and Inflammation in Children and Adolescents: A Systematic Review." *Critical Reviews in Food Science and Nutrition* 60, no. 4 (February 21, 2020): 660–69. https://doi.org/10.1080/10408398 .2018.1546671.

Forrest, Kimberly Y.Z., et al. "Prevalence and Correlates of Vitamin D Deficiency in US Adults." *Nutrition Research* 31, no. 1 (January 2011): 48–54.https://doi.org/10.1016/j .nutres.2010.12.001.

Gennari, Luigi. "Low Vitamin D Levels Independently Associated with Severe COVID-19 Cases, Death." *Endocrine Today*, September 11, 2020. https://www.healio .com/news/endocrinology/20200911/low-vitamin-d-levels-independently-associated -with-severe-covid19-cases-death.

Grant, William B., et al. "Evidence That Vitamin D Supplementation Could Reduce Risk of Influenza and COVID-19 Infections and Deaths." *Nutrients* 12, no. 4 (April 2, 2020): 988. https://doi.org/10.3390/nu12040988.

Lu, Z., Chen, T. C., et al. "An Evaluation of the Vitamin D3 Content in Fish: Is the Vitamin D Content Adequate to Satisfy the Dietary Requirement for Vitamin D?" *The Journal of Steroid Biochemistry and Molecular Biology* 103, no. 3–5 (March 2007): 642–44. https://doi.org/10.1016/j.jsbmb.2006.12.010.

Martineau, Adrian R., et al. "Vitamin D for the Management of Asthma." Edited by Cochrane Airways Group. *Cochrane Database of Systematic Reviews*, September 5, 2016. https://doi.org/10.1002/14651858.CD011511.pub2.

Martineau, Adrian R., et al. "Vitamin D Supplementation to Prevent Acute Respiratory Tract Infections: Systematic Review and Meta-Analysis of Individual Participant Data." *BMJ*, February 15, 2017, i6583. https://doi.org/10.1136/bmj.i6583.

Roy, Satyajeet, et al. "Correction of Low Vitamin D Improves Fatigue: Effect of Correction of Low Vitamin D in Fatigue Study (EViDiF Study)." *North American Journal of Medical Sciences* 6, no. 8 (2014): 396. https://doi.org/10.4103/1947-2714.139291.

Sahota, O. "Understanding Vitamin D Deficiency." *Age and Ageing* 43, no. 5 (September 1, 2014): 589–91. https://doi.org/10.1093/ageing/afu104.

Urashima, Mitsuyoshi, et al. "Randomized Trial of Vitamin D Supplementation to Prevent Seasonal Influenza A in Schoolchildren." *The American Journal of Clinical Nutrition* 91, no. 5 (May 1, 2010): 1255–60. https://doi.org/10.3945/ajcn.2009.29094.

Yang, Chen-Yen, et al. "The Implication of Vitamin D and Autoimmunity: A Comprehensive Review." *Clinical Reviews in Allergy & Immunology* 45, no. 2 (October 2013): 217–26. https://doi.org/10.1007/s12016-013-8361-3.

WHOLE FOOD SUPPLEMENTS

Chapple, Iain L. C., et al. "Adjunctive Daily Supplementation with Encapsulated Fruit, Vegetable and Berry Juice Powder Concentrates and Clinical Periodontal Outcomes: A Double-blind RCT." *Journal of Clinical Periodontology* 39, no. 1 (January 2012): 62–72. https://doi.org/10.1111/j.1600-051X.2011.01793.x.

De Spirt, S., et al. "An Encapsulated Fruit and Vegetable Juice Concentrate Increases Skin Microcirculation in Healthy Women." *Skin Pharmacology and Physiology* 25, no. 1 (2012): 2–8. https://doi.org/10.1159/000330521.

Jin, Yu, et al. "Systemic Inflammatory Load in Humans Is Suppressed by Consumption of Two Formulations of Dried, Encapsulated Juice Concentrate." *Molecular Nutrition &*

Food Research 54, no. 10 (October 2010): 1506–14. https://doi.org/10.1002 /mnfr.200900579.

Kiefer, Ingrid, et al. "Supplementation with Mixed Fruit and Vegetable Juice Concentrates Increased Serum Antioxidants and Folate in Healthy Adults." *Journal of the American College of Nutrition* 23, no. 3 (June 2004): 205–11. https://doi.org/10.1080 /07315724.2004.10719362.

Roll, Stephanie, et al. "Reduction of Common Cold Symptoms by Encapsulated Juice Powder Concentrate of Fruits and Vegetables: A Randomised, Double-Blind, Placebo-Controlled Trial." *British Journal of Nutrition* 105, no. 1 (January 14, 2011): 118–22. https://doi.org/10.1017/S000711451000317X.

ZINC

Alexander, Jan et al. "Early Nutritional Interventions with Zinc, Selenium and Vitamin D for Raising Anti-Viral Resistance Against Progressive COVID-19." *Nutrients* 12, no. 8 (August 7, 2020): 2358. https://doi.org/10.3390/nu12082358.

Black, M. M. "Zinc Deficiency and Child Development." *The American Journal of Clinical Nutrition* 68, no. 2 (August 1, 1998): 464S-469S. https://doi.org/10.1093/ajcn/68 .2.464S.

Heyneman, Catherine A. "Zinc Deficiency and Taste Disorders." *Annals of Pharmacotherapy* 30, no. 2 (February 1996): 186–87. https://doi. org/10.1177/106002809603000215.

Lazzerini, Marzia, and Humphrey Wanzira. "Oral Zinc for Treating Diarrhoea in Children." Edited by Cochrane Infectious Diseases Group. *Cochrane Database of Systematic Reviews*, December 20, 2016. https://doi.org/10.1002/14651858.CD005436. pub5.

Sandstead, H. H. "Understanding Zinc: Recent Observations and Interpretations." *The Journal of Laboratory and Clinical Medicine* 124, no. 3 (September 1994): 322–27.

Solomons, Noel W. "Mild Human Zinc Deficiency Produces an Imbalance Between Cell-Mediated and Humoral Immunity." *Nutrition Reviews* 56, no. 1 (April 27, 2009): 27–28. https://doi.org/10.1111/j.1753-4887.1998.tb01656.x.

Wessels, Inga, et al. "The Potential Impact of Zinc Supplementation on COVID-19 Pathogenesis." *Frontiers in Immunology* 11 (July 10, 2020): 1712. https://doi.org/10.3389 /fimmu.2020.01712.

index

about the author

SHEILA KILBANE, MD, IS a board-certified pediatrician trained in integrative medicine. She is the founder and medical director of Infinite Health, her private practice in Charlotte, North Carolina. Her team of professionals is trained and dedicated to using the best of both conventional and integrative medicine to identify and treat the root cause of children's illnesses.

Based on years of working with thousands of pediatric patients, Dr. Kilbane developed the 7-step program she shares in this book. Her method helps children with chronic or recurrent illnesses achieve significant improvements or complete resolution. An online companion course to this book is available through Dr. Kilbane's website, for families who do not have access to an integrative pediatrician.

Dr. Kilbane is on a mission to transform pediatric healthcare and get one million kids off medications they may not need. Her favorite part of working with families is seeing the light come back into parents' eyes once their child is out of crisis mode—that's when belly laughter can find its place in the home once again.

To help spread the word about how profoundly nutrition impacts children's health, she presents at medical conferences and online summits, and guest blogs and regularly appears on wellness podcasts. She consults with healthcare professionals around the globe as they learn to incorporate integrative medicine into their practices.

Dr. Kilbane splits her time between Charlotte, North Carolina, and Seattle, Washington. She loves just about any outdoor activity with family and friends, and especially enjoys her eight nieces and nephews.